COLLECTED WORKS OF
CHARLES BERG

Volume 5

I0094772

BEING LIVED BY
MY LIFE

BEING LIVED BY MY LIFE

A Sort of Autobiography

CHARLES BERG

R Routledge
Taylor & Francis Group

LONDON AND NEW YORK

First published in 1957 by George Allen & Unwin Ltd

This edition first published in 2022
by Routledge
4 Park Square, Milton Park, Abingdon, Oxon OX14 4RN

and by Routledge
605 Third Avenue, New York, NY 10158

Routledge is an imprint of the Taylor & Francis Group, an informa business

British Library Cataloguing in Publication Data
A catalogue record for this book is available from the British Library

ISBN: 978-1-032-16970-5 (Set)
ISBN: 978-1-003-25348-8 (Set) (ebk)
ISBN: 978-1-032-17129-6 (Volume 5) (hbk)
ISBN: 978-1-032-17137-1 (Volume 5) (pbk)
ISBN: 978-1-003-25194-1 (Volume 5) (ebk)

DOI: 10.4324/9781003251941

Publisher's Note
The publisher has gone to great lengths to ensure the quality of this reprint but points out that some imperfections in the original copies may be apparent.

Disclaimer
The publisher has made every effort to trace copyright holders and would welcome correspondence from those they have been unable to trace.

This book is a re-issue originally published in 1948. The language used is a reflection of its era and no offence is meant by the Publishers to any reader by this re-publication.

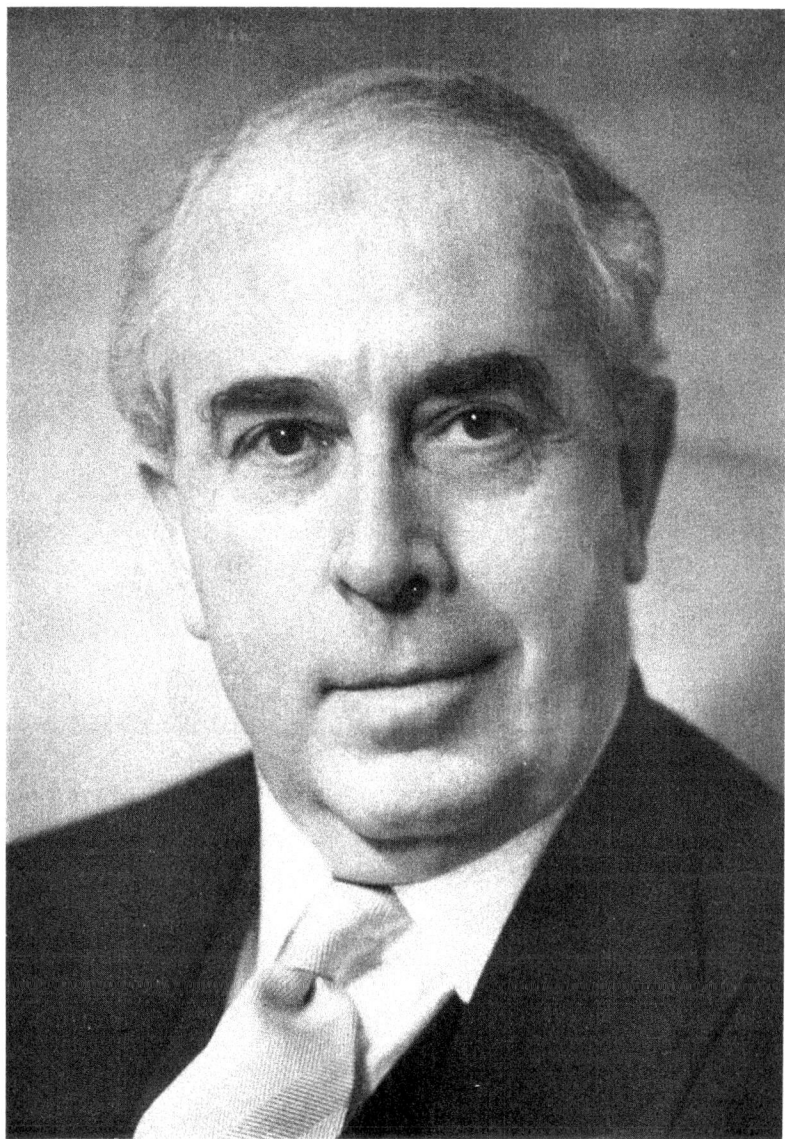

[*photo: Bassano*

THE AUTHOR

CHARLES BERG

Being Lived
by
My Life

A SORT OF AUTOBIOGRAPHY

Ruskin House
GEORGE ALLEN & UNWIN LTD
MUSEUM STREET LONDON

*Printed in Great Britain
in 11 point Bell type
by C. Tinling & Co., Ltd.
Liverpool, London and Prescot*

*My purpose is to display to my kind a
portrait in every way true to nature, and
the man I shall portray will be myself.*

Jean Jacques Rousseau
CONFESSIONS

Myself when young did eagerly frequent
Doctor and Saint, and heard great Argument
        About it and about: but evermore
Came out by the same door as in I went.

With them the Seed of Wisdom did I sow,
And with my own hand laboured it to grow:
        And this was all the Harvest that I reap'd

                            Omar Khayyam

Alas, for me! For I have wandered far,
Past other planets, ringed and bemooned,
Into the starry solitudes of night;
Through chilly darknesses I have been led
By a pale, silent woman, naméd Thought,
To gaze on worlds, lone, uninhabited,
See life evolve from aether, multiply,
And struggle out upon the humid land,
A curious but a very little thing.
I've seen these disappear, and have known
A stillness such that time has ceased to be
And space itself has vanished.
                            Now I stand
Like a bereavéd lover, sick at heart,
Knowing all worlds but as the dust of space
Blown out across a wilderness of time,
And life more fleeting than the tiniest breath,
Breathing within this mighty hurricane
That howls Oblivion.
                            C.B.

With acknowledgements to my son
Adrian Berg
for abridging the original
manuscript of this book

CONTENTS

CHAPTER I

HOLIDAY IN POLZEATH

W H E N my wife broached the question of summer holidays I replied with the now familiar protests: But why arrange and actually *plan* to waste one's time. Wasn't it bad enough that in spite of one's planning *not* to waste one's time, so many hours of waste crept in to the daily industrious programme? There were dozens of things that I wanted to do and ought to do, and could not find time to do, at least not in adequate measure. There were all those books I wanted to write, and had only feebly attempted and rarely completed. What writer or artist is ever satisfied with his work? He always thinks that given time and opportunity, he could or might produce something really good, really worth while. I knew I had not done anything of the sort, and here was my wife talking about summer holidays and planning to waste one's time!

My wife's patience in putting up with this puerile nonsense of mine was finally rewarded by the thought: why not combine the two ideas; let her and the rest of the family have their holiday, while I, though accompanying them, spend the time usefully, writing a book.

No sooner had such a plan taken shape in my mind than it began to mature and no less than a dozen books emerged in embryo. There was, of course, that *magnum opus* (the bête noir of every writer or would-be writer) for which notes had been accumulating for the last thirty years or more, and had even at one stage been filed in an enormous concertina, quite unmanageable in every sense. Then there were volumes of scribble, comprising innumerable 'serial stories-with-a-difference', each 'serial story' the psychological life-history of some anonymous individual, a particular patient of mine, mostly with daily contributions.

However, another one of the long series of projected literary efforts had been suggested to me when a friend had said: 'You yourself have had one of the most varied and complicated existences of any person I have met. Instead of writing little case sheets about these beloved patients of yours, why don't you write an autobiography, a long paper about the star "patient" in your constellation?

You will then have all the psychoses as well as all the neuroses under one skin in one super case-book!'

Born in the Himalayas, in an almost unknown, and now obsolete, little military station hidden miles away amongst the Simla Hills, dragged about the world backwards and forwards from Asia to Europe, round the oceans, all over India, all over Europe, all over London, a hundred and one different schools, never knowing whence I came nor where I was going—surely that alone, even without its chaotic, psychological accompaniment, would make, to say the least of it, an unusual book.

I must confess that all these schemes and several others were still struggling for precedence in my mind when the date arranged for the holiday overtook us. How could it be otherwise? My daily life consists in the customary struggle with the timetable, but perhaps I may say that my particular timetable is hardly customary. It begins at eight or nine a.m. and commonly finishes at eleven p.m. with very small intervals for meals. This does not mean that I am the victim of unending and disagreeable stresses and strains. On the contrary, I sit in a chair, well upholstered (it needs to be) and am entertained, hour by hour, by a succession of serial entertainments of a more interesting nature to me than anybody could obtain by mere payment. What is more, the joke of it is that I get adequately, if not richly, paid for being interested. Of course, awkward and even uncomfortable moments and occasions do arise, but is that not so in every human relationship, even at its best? I may say that it has completely spoilt me for all other pleasures. How can one go on holiday and sit in the lounge of an hotel and listen to old gentlemen, or even young ladies, pouring out their conventionally restricted ideas or, I should say more truthfully, entertaining one to a display of their resistances, when in the comfort of one's home and one's own consulting room one is in the habit of being paid to listen to the less restricted outpourings of the soul, and at the same time nurse the not entirely illusionary satisfaction that one is helping, or being of some use, in so doing.

So a hotel it was not to be, but a home away from home, a home where I could reverse the process of absorbing other people's thoughts and emotions all day long, and instead indulge in the expression of my own . . . if it were possible that there could be an audience that would care to listen.

Anyhow, here we are just arrived at Polzeath, with the prospect of three weeks' interruption of the regular timetable, and the thought has occurred to me that I am on holiday, and therefore why not give myself a real holiday, a holiday from all this psychological and analytical orientation towards individuals and the world, just be a 'patient' myself and simply say whatever I happen to be thinking and feeling. Who can tell what will come of it, if anything. Hence I am calling my initial attempt 'Holiday in Polzeath'.

My experience is that nothing develops so well as freedom of thought and freedom of expression. In fact, the interest and speed of development is directly proportionate to the degree of freedom, the absence of defensive restrictions. If, and this is the doubtful point, I can believe that my audience may be sufficiently sympathetic to warrant it, and if I can in consequence throw aside customary defences and resistances, I may produce something, if not as startling as that which my patients produce in the confines of the analytical chamber, at least something which is some part of the truth, may be a greater part than we are accustomed to reading in print.

Autobiographies commonly begin with a short history of the subject's ancestors, parents and other members of his family, and proceed to describe his birth, childhood and development. I am wondering if this is not an artificial and unnatural method of procedure. Of course, one meets people daily, particularly perhaps neurotic people, whose childhood and antecedents are extraordinarily vivid and intensely interesting. Probably I could fill books with items of vivid experiences of childhood and even of infancy. I am referring to those of *other* people. In my own case, possibly because I am not sufficiently psychoneurotic, I usually find the present moment or something very near to it of primary interest. Therefore if I write naturally, I shall start with the present time. Whether or not it will lead to revivals of the past, remains to be seen. However, there may be an element of novelty in starting now and seeing if the past is contained in the present as so many philosphers and scientists tell us. The present, besides having the advantage of vividness and the absence of the usual nostalgias, has also the advantage, I am tempted to add the very questionable advantage, of being a holiday.

I say questionable because I do think that there may after all be some, however hidden, advantage in holidays. Do I not spend a

certain part of my time trying to convince patients during consultations and sessions that they should, above all, relax their mind
and give themselves a holiday from their customary resistances,
defences and tensions. I tell them that by artifice and effort they
will achieve only a distortion of the truth, whereas nature, the
natural mental processes left to themselves, will produce everything that is true and worthwhile. An objection I sometimes hear is:
'I am afraid I will bore you, doctor'. The answer is that if it is left to
nature nothing will be boring, nature never bores, only subter-
fuges or blanketings of anxiety-driven man. It is when nature is
covered up or substituted by something relatively false that we are
bored. Reality, truth and nature cannot bore. Thus, if I can really
succeed in letting my mind take a holiday, a natural process may
reveal itself which should avoid the tediousness of the orthodox
autobiographical writing. Is such a thing possible? Having drilled
myself for so many years to be the paid observer while other
people's minds take a holiday, having grown accustomed almost
all my waking hours, to be on duty in this way, I may find it impossible to reverse the process and give myself, particularly my mind,
the sort of holiday I advocate for others. Have I become too much of
a machine in the analytical laboratory to be able to 'take my place
in nature?' I have often said that to do analysis is, or becomes, an
all-or-nothing process. Either one is steeped in it more or less to
the exclusion of all else, or, if anything of the outside world in-
trudes, even the *prospect* of an imminent holiday, away goes one's
capacity as an analyst. Maybe one cannot live in two worlds at the
same time, that of the unconscious levels of the mind, and that of
the conscious substitutive realities around one, especially if these
latter are going to insist upon the distraction of one's attention.

Thus, having arrived at this beautiful little place in Cornwall
with its deep estuary and its valley-beach, sheltered by the surrounding hills, one's first tendency is to wonder why one is here,
what is the sense in it, and what is it all about. I shall resist the
temptation to talk about my surroundings, the things *outside* me, as
so many patients do when they don't like the things *inside*, and
want to avoid talking about them. It is what we call 'resistance',
and if I am going to resist why bother to write at all. In writing
about myself in the first person, I realise that I am laying myself
open to all the ribald criticisms that rude (in the old English

sense) men and women delight in, but then what does it matter? I realise also that I am growing old (who is not; the one certain thing about every living organism is that it must die—though not one of us really believes this of himself) and who am I to deny any person, rude or otherwise, his delight! I have lived long enough and have listened long enough to sufficient people on the analytical settee to be convinced that those who place their highest value on civilisation and conventional attitudes are worshipping the golden calf, false gods; but I am not going to break my tablets on their account nor on any other account. Civilisation and convention have their value, but it is a limited, defensive and substitutive value. It covers the truth of which we are afraid and offers substitutes for it. Most people conceal the truth within them for fear of derision, even those under analysis do this for a long time, but not entirely, and not for ever. Perhaps the best compliment that can be paid to me, or to anybody, is derision! I am resolved that I shall in these pages try my best not to stoop to any stunt form of writing, nor shall I consciously even attempt to be humorous. The only constant guide shall be none other than that which I daily and hourly never tire of advocating, namely unadulterated naturalness. By that alone I will sink or swim. I have come to the conclusion after a long life that it is better even to sink being natural, than to perfom extraordinary feats at the sacrifice of being oneself.

CHAPTER II

GENESIS

I F there is one thing that is emerging from these deliberations, it is the thesis of naturalness as a principle. I owe my belief in this to more than one source, to more than one particular series of experiences. First amongst these must be placed my analytical and psychotherapeutic orientation and clinical experience. A practical exponent is my now-adult son. He, like other individualists I have known, seems to take without question that being himself is a *sine quo non* of his existence. If I say to him: 'But you will earn ten times the income as a doctor,' or 'Why don't you have a fourth year at Cambridge and become a don?' he replies simply: 'Because I shall paint.' That is all there is to it. The point is that to paint is him, and, live or die, painting (i.e. himself) naturally has not only precedence over everything, but is indissolubly bound up with him as part and parcel of his very existence, of his *raison d'être*. So naturalness it is. 'For what shall it profit a man if he shall gain the whole world and lose his own soul?' If a man sacrifices naturalness, or in so far as he sacrifices naturalness, he loses that much of himself, of his very life. At the best he will suffer for his pains internal stresses and strains, whether or not these emerge as symptoms, psychoneurotic, psychosomatic or organic, characterological, national or international. (I hope all this will be explained as this work or play unfolds.) Even symptoms, not to mention characterological peculiarities, may be preferable to internal tensions unrelieved—or so Nature seems to think.

I am reminded of the story I have often told against one of our top-notch psychiatrists. At a particularly pretentious seminar at the Royal Society of Medicine, Dr. Top-Notch boasted at great length about the large number of psychoneurotic patients cured annually at his enormous mental out-patient department. Thereupon a true psychologist amongst us arose and asked naïvely whether the great doctor really thought it necessary to deprive all those poor sufferers of their only means of relieving their tensions! Maybe it was more natural for them and maybe more comfortable, more consistent with health, to have their symptoms than to learn to suppress them.

Symptoms only disappear healthily when a re-adjustment or new distribution of energy is made within the mind which enables the tensions which give rise to them to find an alternative outlet more satisfactory to every level of the mind. Without such a redistribution of psychic energy, it may be more natural for some people to have symptoms than not. Indeed, I hope that a proper assessment of this present work will ultimately enable every reader to appreciate without any shadow of doubt that all the activities of himself, and indeed of everybody including those of mankind as a whole, his civilisation and everything, can be appropriately and scientifically described as 'symptomatic' mental and physical behaviour. That is not to say that it should be suppressed—any more than the symptoms displayed by Dr. Top-Notch's patients should have been suppressed.

Are we already getting a new orientation to the concept of 'cure'? How tired I am of people arriving in my consulting room and asking me if I can cure them. Maybe the trouble with us all is that our life from birth has been an unwarranted agony of being cured. I am convinced by dint of long experience, both in organic medicine and in psychiatry, that all our illnesses, including organic disease of every description, are essentially the fruit of these cures, in some cases extending through a period considerably longer than that of one individual's lifetime. However, do not believe me yet.

It may well be asked what I have to offer, if anything, in exchange for this gratuitous attempt to cure the reader of his symptomatic belief in the concept of cure! Yes indeed, and I think I can vouchsafe an answer. Whatever am I saying? No, I am not claiming that I shall within these pages reveal the complete answer to the riddle of the universe, but I am definitely suggesting that I can make some little contribution to a revelation of the secret of happiness. Well I know that enormous revelations of this secret have been claimed at successive periods through the ages. The secret of happiness has been no less a concern of all than has been the riddle of the universe, but my claim this time has two important differences. One is that it is not large or sweeping, it does not pretend to be more than a very minute suggestion in the right direction. The other is that whatever it achieves or does not achieve, I can promise that it will do so without any sacrifice whatsoever of the truth. In this respect it would certainly be unique. All I can tell you about it at the moment is in the form of a personal testimonial. I myself ordinarily enjoy a greater measure of contentment than most people I have met. Of course, there may be nothing startling or exceptional about this; I have no doubt that there are hundreds, thousands, probably millions of people as contented as, or even more contented than, I can claim to be (no doubt it would not be difficult to point to cows in the field and declare that I had nothing on them!) but, I am inclined to ask, how many of them have been through such a period of restlessness, of strain and endeavour before they learnt it, before they acquired a contentment comparable to mine?

Before I go any further with this boastful claim, I must emphasize that I am as well aware as any of us, I hope, that no living person, organism or blade of grass is separate from or independent of the forces around it, of the natural phenomena that brought it into being, and upon which its condition at any and every moment of its existence directly depends. It would be a sad day for all of us, or it would herald a sad day, if fortune were so unvaringly perfect that we fostered the illusion that we were above or immune from the hazards of fate. Maybe we are all apt to suffer a little from such an illusion, and that is why death is so sad.

With reference to my own personal contentment, I had a recent salutary reminder of its potential instability, and if I had needed anything to correct the analyst's pretence and tendency to pose as superhuman, this effectively assured me that I was no better than other helpless children. I refer to a recent occasion when my infant sustained a severe burn which, up to the third day, I fancied might endanger its health or even its life. Contentment was as though it had never been. There was nothing in the whole universe except one enormous anxiety. However apparently successful the pose one assumes, one has only to encounter some personal insecurity such as illness, death, danger to children, or accident, and down one comes crashing from one's pedestal to be revealed to oneself as not one iota better than one's own worst anxiety-ridden, drug-addicted or psychotic patient.

This should remind us that our qualities or nature, like our very existence or non-existence, our illness or our health, our honesty or our dishonesty, are not matters for which we are justified in claiming any credit, or, to be logical, for that matter discredit. We are nothing more or less than the product of forces around us, the very forces which brought us into being and which take us out of it. How could it be otherwise? It is not our universe. We are merely creatures of it.

Perhaps these considerations put my claim that I can show something of the forces which led to my own personal contentment in its right perspective. The matter of sufficient interest to warrant the telling of the story is the fact that this contentment is an end-product of a life of more than average restlessness. Many stories purport to tell us how tragedy of some sort came about. Others are, perhaps correctly, based upon the painful or stressful symptomatic behaviour or happenings of adolescent or early life being transformed by the biologically sound, if not inevitable, acquisition of a mate; to which event we can add, in spite of the cynics, the very appropriate words: 'Lived happily ever after.'

It is a scientific truth, revealed throughout most analyses, that the pre-mating period is one of id-stress (instinct-stress), the only real and lasting solution of which is achieved by an adequate satisfactory sexual adjustment. Thus, 'Lived happily ever after' should be the only correct 'cure', by appropriate adjustment, of the needs of the instinctual levels which we call the '*id*'. Unfortunately, we have often in the meantime become too morbid for it to be as large a cure as it should be for wants or needs at every level of the mind. It may be that my story goes a little deeper, though I hope it will be just as simple. It purports to show how the contentment, which I now enjoy throughout these years of my life, settled upon me after innumerable stresses and vicissitudes. Was it the fruit of the policy I here advocate, namely the policy of sacrificing everything in favour of the greatest possible naturalness, being 'oneself' above all the riches of man and the promises of God and the Devil? Was it?

What we have at the moment nearer at hand is the matter of this book and the principle I have suggested as essential to its conception, namely to let it unfold naturally, scorning or refusing to build an ego-constructed, i.e. unnatural, framework for it, and still less to allow my ego or superego to construct a 'blue-print' to ensure the usual illusionary success.

I have had to adapt myself to many and various changing realities, or is it that I have been adapted *by* them? Groddeck tells us, and how rightly, that we do not live our lives, but that we are lived by life, by the *'id'* (his word), by the forces that flow into us and through us. Can we let it rest at that, and avoid introducing our anxiety-ridden interferences, our attempted cures, amassed upon that which would be perfectly all right without such artificial nonsense? Nature implanted in the course of evolution, instinct patterns within us. Are these the only guide deserving any confidence? They certainly have the priority in time. They appear to have led to our survivial so far. Attempts at alteration with a view to further adaptation may conceivably be a sign of advancing stages in the process of evolution. We should be very sure that they *are* this before daring to interfere with the laws of nature. We should be sure that they are the necessary adaptation to reality and not just a bit of psychotic nonsense (which they usually are) before we set about increasing our and other people's stresses and endangering the health, nay the very existence and survival, of ourselves and others in the process; for there is no doubt that the one thing we can be sure of in such attempts, the characteristic of civilisation, is a painful and discontented passage from the cradle to the grave.

Is it really necessary to have a compulsive drive? If we look upon life as the brief passage which it is from the cradle to the grave, perhaps comfort and happiness may be valued more than sweat and toil—unless of course we have a compulsive drive that we must relieve or else suffer. If the latter is the case our life may be regarded as the expression of a symptom, an attempt (futile or incompletely successful) to relieve an inner pain or tension.

A virile, dynamic man, a patient of mine, contemplating getting married for the second time, was wondering whether he would get 'fed up' with the quiet life which he envisaged if married to this particular lady. He said: 'When I was married before, and my wife used to sit in her chair and take her knitting out for the evening and I would be expected to read a book, I would look at her quietly and think. . . .' I do not know whether his next remark was what he thought, or an explosive expression of what he was feeling at this moment contemplating the scene—'Christ!' he shouted, 'I might as well be under the ground.' He continued: 'I couldn't stand it. Oh for the liveliness that used to go on in my home when I was a boy! I think I would rather have those terrible rows that I have cursed so loudly, than this. This is like death. The other was at least *alive*.'

Is this man telling us that life without a compulsive drive is, to him at least, not so much contentment as death?

Two reflections emerge from this: one is that if we put a play upon the stage in which there were nothing but contentment, people knitting or reading beside the fireplace, it would surely not be long before the audience yawned a few times, and then walked out. The same would apply to all our novels, stories, conversations, and perhaps to everything else. The importance of the second reflection cannot be over-estimated; I can vouch for its absolute truth, as every hour of my analytical experience goes to reveal it afresh and to verify it again and again. It is the analytical revelation that evey one of us, whether he knows it or not, and he generally does not know it, has a compulsion to repeat throughout his life the emotional patterns which were created and developed in him during the earliest years of his life.

One may go back further than that in phylogenetic evolution, and assert that everyone is compelled to repeat the emotional patterns brought into being long before his birth and inherited by him in the form of instincts. This is well known and accepted, at least it is accepted that we have instincts, but what is not adequately recognised is the truth that there is something created in us between the instinct level and the conscious level, created in our early years, and in a sense more complicated and more closely related to our reality contacts, which analytical experience reveals to us as having a compulsive effect comparable only to that of the instincts, and riding rough-shod over all our so-called realities.

For example, the patient to whom I have referred was brought up in a more than usually turbulent household. There were daily rows between his father and mother, there were hysterical outbursts on her part at almost every meal, sometimes reaching the climax of her rushing from the table in tears, slamming doors and threatening suicide. The effect upon the child witness of all this has to be experienced during his analysis to be believed. He claims to have longed throughout for stability and a peaceful existence; he declares that he used to leave the house as much as possible and play with friends outside in order to avoid these intolerable, turbulent scenes. But what are the effects as seen to-day? He has been left economically secure with every material provision for a peaceful, quiet and happy life, yet the disturbances within him are understandable only in the light of what used to go on in his home during his childhood. Analytically, one experiences samples of it all during his hourly sessions. Instead of peaceful, happy contemplation, contentment in the security of his reality situation, we find a sullen discontent until he gets into his stride, and then we get shouting and rows throughout the time, understandable only in the light of their being reproductions of childhood. They are the only forms of expression which give him relief from an intolerable internal tension.

In short, he is either holding his tensions in and feeling intensely uncomfortable, even physically uncomfortable—he says: 'I can feel my duodenal ulcer forming when I keep quiet, like every other male in our family has had'—or else he is what he calls blowing off, shouting and raving, going off the deep end. However torn he may be during these expressions of himself, they are the only thing that makes him feel better afterwards. Possibly his mother and father also felt better after their rows. It would seem that there is no quiet married life in prospect for him. It would not even feel to him like death; it would feel like agony, an agony which he could not and certainly would not endure. There would be upheavals, shoutings and rows until his second wife fled as his first has already done.

The reason he is not working is because, in his present unanalysed state, such rows would inevitably arise in whatever society he were in and make his employment impossible. Though he has recognised that they are replicas or expressions of the emotions aroused within him in his childhood, emotions which at that time had to be more repressed than they are now, the mere recognition does not cure the tendency. He still suffers intolerable tension unless he can relieve it in this fashion, so accurately identical with the environment of his childhood.

I am here reminded of another patient, an enormous, six-foot-four, physically and mentally powerful man, who tells me that when he heard me in the passage approaching the door of the waiting room to call him for his session, he felt a cold shiver down his spine, broke into a sweat and started to tremble from head to foot. He thought he heard me rattling a stick in the hall outside, and momentarily anticipated that I would enter and lay about him. His association of thought was immediately an infantile memory relating to the age of four when his cruel stepmother, more cruel than any of those in legend (truth is stranger than fiction), used to come up the stairs with a stick, which he had heard her selecting from the hall stand, to beat him unmercifully for his bed-wetting.

It would be a mistake to think that these emotional reactions appear only in the analytical setting. This man has similar reactions to all his employees in his office. Of course, they do not suspect it, for he covers it up, or over-compensates for it, by being the most harsh, bullying employer imaginable. Analysis reveals that in infancy he knew of only two roles in his childhood environment— either that of being the beaten and frightened little boy, or that of being the beating and frightening stepmother. He has to act the latter in order to avoid feeling the former.

There is no difference between emotional reactions in analytical sessions and those which go on in ordinary life. The only difference between the two situations is that in analysis the patient can recognise that he has no reality justification or causation for the way he is feeling and reacting emotionally, whereas in real life he is better able to rationalise his feelings and behaviour, or indeed, usually unconsciously, to engineer or to create reality situations which seem to justify them. In other words, analysis shows that we are all endeavouring to make a world around us which will be suitable, if not appropriate, for the relief of our tensions created by the emotional patterns of our early life.

The closeness of these unconscious mechanisms to instinctual compulsions may be recognisable. The nearest these sufferers, and indeed everyone of us, can get to internal comfort, or shall we call it contentment, is in accordance with their success in creating an environment, a world around them, which lends itself to the natural expression of these ingrained patterns, and thereby enables them to discharge the tensions within, which they otherwise create and accumulate.

Therefore, to say, as some critics of applied psychoanalysis are never tired of saying, that the standard of reality, that the scientific revelations obtained in the consulting-room, specifically during analysis, are in no wise applicable to the wider world of man, is manifestly not entirely true. Indeed, analysis shows us that the 'wider world of man' is in many respects, perhaps in all, a product of the unconscious machinations of the unconscious minds of men in unison, operating through the ages. Resistance to a recognition of this can also be seen operating throughout every analytical session. We all prefer, unless we are neurotic, to live our emotions in the present day, and to nurse the illusion that they belong solely to the present day, as though we had no past. It may be that unless we keep our minds very superficial, concentrated exclusively upon the immediate matters around us, interferences from our would-be forgotten past, especially from childhood, are liable to emerge and to disturb our superficiality. What is liable to do this is not memory, for the conceptual forms of things are all too easily kept from consciousness; it is solely emotional feelings and patterns which, without their relevant memories or concepts, have no meaning for us, and are apt to be merely disturbing or confusing.

I was recently consulted by a young man who found it difficult to formulate his complaint, but got as far as saying that he seemed to be lacking any drive in life and felt that his mind was in a state of confusion. When I asked him how far back in his life he could trace this unsatisfactory mental state, he replied: 'All my life; I remember that I felt very confused as a boy at school. In fact, my mind was chaotic.' During a subsequent interview with his father, when I referred to this remark to indicate the long duration of the trouble, as a counter to the latter's hope that cure would be rapid, the father interestingly dismissed the matter with the remark: 'Well, which of us wasn't confused in his school days? I know I was.'

This remark has caused me to reflect upon my own state of confusion throughout early life, not only at school but even at the university. I think I know something about its causation. It is, I am sure, the result of a defensive process. We are all being unnatural, largely concerned to maintain our unnaturalness at all costs. There is an effort going on within the mind, one might almost call it an effort to be stupid and remain stupid. It is a defensive measure. Probably it has two phases: one is that we are trying to exclude from consciousness the interfering tendency of our repressed emotions, instincts and childhood patterns; the other is that we are so busy doing this, so much mental energy is taken up in the process, that we have perforce similarly to exclude a great deal of the stimulating realities around us. As early as 1920 Freud elucidated a process which he called 'blocking', the blocking from entry into the mind of unwanted or excessive stimulation. This was part of a process called 'primal repression', which led on to the 'binding' of unwanted stimuli which had got past this first defence, and so on to the concept of 'repression' proper. In short, we have to protect our conscious mind from undue interferences, both from within and without, by keeping it, as it were, encased in a protective box of stupidity. The affective consequence of all this, or perhaps the affective consequence of some forces breaking through in spite of all this, is the experience of confusion. In any case, we do not know the source of the feelings we feel, and that in itself is puzzling and confusing.

I see myself now as a wide-eyed, confused infant being carted about the world, as a schoolboy with all those strange and noisy companions around me, perhaps not quite understanding why I had been separated from my mother. I see myself a little later digging in our garden at Villa les Platanes, Lausanne, Switzerland, about fifteen years of age, somewhat at the crossroads of life, not quite understanding what it was all about, where I had come from or where I was going, but knowing that it was important that I should know, at least have some idea of an answer to the latter question. It was even a bit worrying. What was I doing digging in a garden? Somehow, the last year or two had overtaken my parents unawares, and it was discovered that I was too late for an English public school.

I think it was this confusion which was responsible for the idea forming in my mind that I would become a philosopher! After all, the thing of importance was to get some answer to this vague and puzzling question of source, and particularly of destination. So philosophy it would have to be. Of course, I had never thought of bread and butter—that had always been provided, as it is with every dependant, like manna from heaven.

CHAPTER III

SCHOOL AND NEURALGIA

WITH regard to philosophy as a programme, some modifications had had to be made. There was no certain career or future in it. Medicine, on the other hand, gave one entry not only to a definite profession, but also a definite economic career, and I was told I would learn a great deal about the things I wanted to know in the course of pursuing the medical curriculum. Since the experience of doing so, I have always held that an education in medicine is a very important, perhaps an essential basis for any and every education. This applies particularly to the first year of study; how could one ever begin to understand the universe or anything without a preliminary knowledge of physics, chemistry and biology. But it was not these subjects that puzzled me; on the contrary, they were delightfully revealing and I might even say reassuring. What did puzzle me was the nature and behaviour of all the people, particularly the young people, the undergraduates, around me. I fancy that schoolboys may have puzzled me even more, but the mystery of the world of schoolboys was in all essentials continued in the mystery of the world of these young men.

Two of my closest associates happened to be Roman Catholics. I cannot describe the puzzlement created in my mind on the one hand by the fact of their religious beliefs, and, on the other hand by the completely irrelevant and equally incomprehensible fact of their emotions and behaviour. How many separate and irreconcilable compartments there must be in the human mind when one reflects that one at least of these monkey-like young men was also a brilliant scholar. It will be seen that I yet had a great deal to learn outside the department of physics, chemistry and biology. I may add that I am now far from convinced that one department is outside another.

The important point I wish to stress in regard to these many years in medical school and hospital, particularly medical school, is that in spite of the background of confusion, everything was not entirely chaotic; perhaps one had to have some integrative thread to guide one through the maze. One certainly had more than a thread; there was a drive into which was drawn or forced every available scrap of energy and enthusiasm that one could muster to further its purpose. It might well be that one was at a loss regarding the purpose or destiny of man, including oneself. In a large or wide sense, one was all at sea regarding an ultimate purpose and direction. But there was one immediate purpose, one immediate direction about which one could have no doubt, and that was the purpose of mastering the mysteries of the scientific subjects presented to one and the putting aside of anything and everything, particularly internal things, that tended to interfere with that purpose; and they were surely more abundant and forceful than any of us realized.

However, by dint of all the endeavour of which the energy and vigour of youth is capable, one even succeeded to some extent in creating a God, or idol that had the appearances of a God, in mustering an extraordinary degree of real, positive enthusiasm. I mean one engendered even some emotional element in the positive pioneering in this unknown country. If it were not the riddle of the universe that one was solving, it had at least something to do with it It was little bits or aspects of the universe carefully separated from the larger issues and presented for specialised and detailed attention. The thing might fit together in the end and form an understandable picture, and then perhaps the riddle would be solved and this unsatisfactory state of confusion brought to and end.

After all, was I so far from my original ambition of philosophy? These sciences were even called natural philosophy, and clearly a knowledge of them was essential to anything and everything. I found later, having passed through relatively interminable years of detailed specialisation—anatomy, physiology, midwifery, gynaecology, children, pathology, medicine, surgery, fevers, skins, ear, nose and throat, etc. ctc.—that my original addiction to philosophy re-asserted itself, it had never disappeared. The problem that remained unsolved throughout the medical curriculum, the problem which was presented to one, this time with even practical importance, was again the problem of people, really the problem of oneself projected and extended. All these people that one saw in general practice, whether they had illnesses of their organs, skins, or ear, throat or nose, all had essentially a much bigger problem, the same problem that one had onself, namely their problem as a person, the problem of their source, destiny, or rather what concerned them more consciously, the problem of their feelings and emotions and mental state. Whether they knew it or not, it was easy to see that they were fundamentally as confused as I was. Also, I felt sure that all these minor and major troubles, of which they complained, were only distractions; the fundamental problem was far more important than all these. Nevertheless, all were undoubtedly related.

A not uninteresting aspect of all this was the problem of the apparatus which was all we had, all that we could bring to bear upon this enormous aspect or portion of the riddle of the universe. I became more and more convinced, as philosophers had done thousands of years before me, that these two subjects were complementary and indissolubly connected, namely the subject of the instrument and the subject of the object. Originally, both were included under the term philosophy, psychology being the name for that which concerned itself with the instrument, ontology the name for that half of philosophy which directed its attention to the universe outside the mind. No doubt they were only apparently distinct ways of looking at the same thing.

There is an important omission in the course of this reference to the history of my life, an omission which it will not do to ignore entirely, as it is surely most relevant to the theoretical structure and understanding which I anticipate will eventually emerge from these deliberations. It must be an integral part of the whole psychopathology of my developing adjustment, internal and external. The omission to which I refer is—you may be surprised to hear it—trigeminal neuralgia. I am sure it was intimately bound up with scholastic endeavour, or rather with the stresses and strains, the effortful repressions contingent upon that endeavour.

I can still remember the occasion when it was suddenly borne home to me that I was not exactly as other men are (!) or rather as other boys of ten years around me at the time were. I was at a funny little school, sitting in an incredibly funny little classroom, one of a line perched against a steep hill-side in a rather remote part of the Mussoorie hills. I had come to that school nearly at the end of term, and we had just completed the end-of-term examinations. There were only about twelve boys in my class. Somebody asked the woman teacher who was going to be first. She looked towards me, and laughed, and said: 'He's different.' Different, me different! *Of course* I was different. Why was I different? Because nobody but me had *my mother* as his mother. Nobody else had my mother behind him, my mother who was so alive to every thought and feeling that I had or might have, my mother who was so emotionally alive to every hair of my head, to every fibre of my being. What a tower of strength behind little me! They did not know, they could have no idea, that I lived in a citadel of mother-love, of mother-power, that was proof against all the slings and arrows . . . against the whole world of small boys and big men, against the universe, a citadel against which the cosmos would beat in vain. I was brought up in an atmosphere of such security and love that I could develop naturally, that I could be just exactly myself, without any fear. I knew without any shadow of doubt that I myself would be accepted by my mother without any diminution of her love. This is the sense of security that every child needs.

Sometime later when, through over-crowding, we were studying in the prefects' classroom, I remember that the head prefect—monitors they called them in that school—expressed incredulity with great emphasis, and then turned round and, staring hard at me, said 'Good God!' Apparently his conviction that I was half-witted had received a grave shock in the light of some newly acquired information. The same sort of thing happened in school after school, conspicuously in the larger school at Simla a year later. Mentally I must have been at least two years above my class age; I had no work to do, except to correct the mathematical papers of the rest of the class as our science teacher from Cambridge claimed to have no knowledge of mathematics and delegated me to do his work while he read a book at the desk. I did not seem to have to study at all. I have no doubt that had I been put in a class two years higher I would still have been first, but at that age I was, of course, very content to rest on my easily won laurels. There was no scholastic endeavour, but I am sure the stresses were already there in the mind. I am inclined to think that they were more inherited than acquired. So far as acquired factors are concerned, I am sure that it was no more than a descreditable cowardice, in fact an acute, unreasonable fear of the teacher, of the boys, and of the publicity of making an exhibition of myself and

of my fear. It was the intensity of this morbid fear that caused my
mind to be constantly alert, as it were on its toes all the time, and
which mobilised every one of my faculties, as fear does, to miss
nothing and to bring every ounce of intelligence that I could muster
to bear upon the situation. It was a defensive mobilisation and intense activity of mind focused upon the reality dangers.

I think this process must have started very early in life, for by
the age that I have recently referred to, when I was teaching the
class mathematics, I was already reaping the benefit of this previous
stimulation and development, and finding myself intellectually
above my contemporaries. There was therefore perhaps small
wonder that I began to compensate myself for my frustrations,
perhaps for my internal stresses, by nursing the phantasy, the fond
illusion, that I was some special creation of nature, designed to
answer all the riddles and to solve all the problems which the
inadequate minds of other men had not yet succeeded in doing.
The enlightenment of man was awaiting my maturity. It seemed
I was to be a Messiah, the coming intellectual Messiah! Some may
think that I richly deserved the agonies which were soon to over-
take me and puncture my smug anticipations.

The point of psychopathological interest is that I feel the precursors of neuralgia were already there. Though commonly healthy,
I can remember periodic bouts of strange feelings, both locally in
the head and generally. There was some migrainous diathesis that
was soon to make itself felt as periodic, acute trigeminal neuralgia.
This wretched complaint dogged my footsteps throughout the
greater half of my life, right up to the time that I was psycho-
analysed. It was a black cloud that used to descend upon me
practically without warning in the course of my serious intellectual
pursuits, and apparently without any ascertainable or avoidable
cause. It would come suddenly, out of the bluest sky, and would
recur daily with increasing severity for days or weeks. It would
reach a pitch that was quite unendurable; but when it passed, one's
tendency was to forget that it ever occurred, and to pick up the
threads of one's life again.

Of course, I saw occasional, though rare, cases of similar trouble
referred to hospital. I still remember the young woman in my later
student days when surgical dresser, who came in and had her
Gasserian ganglion on the left side removed. I studied her thought-

fully; her case was worse than mine. She was eager for any operation. Had it been proposed to remove both eyes, nose or everything else, she would have gladly assented in the hope that these attacks of hers would be cured. Any portion of her brain she would willingly have sacrificed; in fact, I think she would have assented most enthusiastically to the certain cure of decapitation. She knew, as I knew, what the surgical proposals meant. Fortunately, that form of ghastly operation is, I believe, obsolete. Perhaps the time will come when all operations for neuralgia are obsolete. I watched this young woman recover; I observed the facial paralysis, the sewing-up of the lids of her left eye to prevent the corneal ulceration which tended to follow; I watched the shocking disfigurement that remained on her previously pretty face . . . and in due course I observed that she still got her trigeminal neuralgia, although it seemed every possible physical basis for it had been removed. One can best explain it on the analogy of the pain a person can get in even the big toe of a leg that has been amputated. The essential receptive cells in the nervous system and in the Cortex of the brain are, of course, still there, and still impressed with the stimuli that apparently once used to reach them. In the case of neuralgia, it may well be that it is the receptive cells in the central nervous system which are the primary trouble, the pain in them being only referred to their peripheral supply. Thus one would be removing a part that is quite irrelevant to the pain.

The reason I have had to mention neuralgia is not only on account of its psychological relevance to the great drive and endeavour of my student years, but also because I feel that the tensions lying at the root of that drive were, even in childhood, related to the tensions which produced the agonising pain. Probably the whole of life throughout those many years, until ripe maturity at least, was basically an agony of which I had little or no conscious conception. I do not think this is entirely a contradiction in terms; I am sure that enormous stresses can remain unconscious and liable to reveal themselves along paths other than those of consciousness. I think practically all organic disease owes its origin to some such process. Of course, the unconscious agony, tied up as it were in the deeper levels of the mind, may still reach consciousness by these devious organic routes, with or without some direct breaking through repression into the conscious levels. All such agony, or if we do not like the use of a term like agony, which usually implies something conscious, let us say all unconscious strains or tensions denote nervous or psychic energy which is not finding the normal path along which to discharge itself. The experience of the discharge of psychic tension along an unrestricted or uninhibited path, accompanied as it is by a usually conscious feeling of relief, is probably the very essence of the sensation which we call pleasure, whether the mechanisms involved are simple, primitive, inherited paths, or whether they are complicated, multiple structures involving many levels of the psyche.

Now, all this talk of tension, scholarship and neuralgia has its point. It tells me that under the guidance or misguidance of my well-meaning environment—civilisation, father, mother and everyone—I was being caused, or the nature within me, unable to use the facilities offered adequately, was causing me movement towards an intolerable, increasing amount of pain. As I have said, either the environment was odd or phoney, or I (the ingredients of me) was odd or phoney; at any rate, the one did not fit the other. Instead of being comfortable, natural and contented, I was accumulating strain, tension and potential agony. Have I not seen a similar picture in almost every person I have studied, patient or so-called normal? However, there is a variation in intensity and degree of this trouble. Perhaps it is the primitive animal being forced into the unfitting or mis-shapen iron hat or straitjacket of civilisation. We may return to that subject later. As when the steam pressure within a boiler is continually increasing, and either the wheels are not being allowed to go fast enough, or the safety valves discharge themselves, or for some other reason pressure is steadily increasing beyond the means of discharge, so with the human psyche must something sooner or later happen. In the case of the boiler, obviously an explosion; in the case of the organism developed biologically, perhaps the best thing that can happen is a re-activation, a re-opening of some previously closed, civilisation-closed channel for discharge. Many abnormal consequences, atavistic and otherwise, are thus rendered possible; a human organism may burst open at its least well-sealed points.

There is, however, one normal channel through which they all burst. If they do not, or do not do so adequately, some abnormality, negative if not positive, will sooner or later assert itself. What

I wish to say here, though, is that the intensity or degree of the outburst, however normal in kind, varies considerably from one individual to another. Maybe some were destined by nature, though evidently not by man or by civilisation, to continue the species, and others to fade out by the wayside in a few generations, if not immediately.

The occasion often arises at an analytical session, especially with a very genuine and emotionally dynamic analysand, when the patient suddenly gives vent to an outburst of impatience with all the stuff and nonsense that he or the analyst has been talking, and comes out explosively with his pent-up emotions in their naked or nascent form.

I had a patient the other day who blathered politely and reasonably for fifteen minutes, showing signs of rising tension and increasing restlessness all the time he did so, and then suddenly yelled: 'To hell with all this hooey! The fact is I'm sick of it. I don't want this cold slab (analysis). I'm hot with anger. I don't want any more politeness; I'm full of hate, hate of all sloppy good manners and politeness and feebleness. I want to shout louder (he was yelling). It's the healthiness in me that's bloody angry. I ought to come and smash everything up.'

Now, a similar thing to this patient's first quarter-hour has been taking place in the writing of these would-be free-associations of thought; the ego has done a lot of talking, a lot of covering up. Maybe that has been necessary, at least as a preliminary; perhaps our natures, our psychology, or even our *physiology* do not permit us to get straight down to the essentials of anything, particularly of feelings or emotions. . . . Life itself may be a waste of time between its two or three important events. Perhaps important events could not be important unless there were a sort of build-up in advance, there could not be an explosion unless there were a resistant encasement built around the explosive material. But I think the true analogy is a little different from all these. It is this: there could not be an orgasm unless there were a preliminary accumulation of psychosexual tension. Every outburst of energy requires some energy to have accumulated preparatory to the bursting out. Perhaps that is why patients cannot be cured psychologically in one session; the whole process has to go through a succession of stages. If we started by interpreting the root of the

C

trouble we would only shock the patient into firmer resistance, in fact he might place more than a resistance between himself and us— he might place a considerable amount of space! Therapy must be done in stages. We must first seem to be part of, to side with, the patient's ego structure, however full it may be of resistance. It is only after he has identified us with his accepted superficial levels that we will be in a position, that we will have gained his confidence sufficiently, to give him courage to open some of the hidden and sealed up places.

Well, such is my excuse for having built up these chapters of writing on what I would call a more or less ego-acceptable basis. I may, nevertheless, have roused resistance on the part of many readers; some of course will never touch the book at all; others would soon put it down, even in the earliest chapters having come across something, or much, that was contrary to their conventional or accepted tenets. I must apologise only to those who have tended to put it down through being impatient with me for such an elaborate build-up of defences, those who were ready and who wanted to come to grips with essential and important matters right away, or at least at an earlier stage than this. However, I have many excuses. I have noticed how appraisal from the public, including educated critics who should know better, is given analytical authors in direct proportion to the length and elaborateness of their ego-constructed cover, and how commonly or usually abuse and vituperations fall upon anyone, in relation to the extent, and particularly to the suddenness, with which he reveals the naked truth.

I have spoken at length of many sloppy emotions and concepts: contentment, naturalness, intellectualism, highly constructed, sublimated drives, the emotional force behind an urge to discover, to solve, the riddle of oneself and the riddle of the universe. I may even have given the impression that this drive was the power of my life that led me through some moderate degree of scholastic achievement towards philosophy. I have referred also to stresses and pain and agony. What I have carefully concealed is joy, joy that was more powerful than all the intellectual structures and sublimations, joy that swept aside everything including pain, joy that was and is the real dynamic force which is life, and without which life has no meaning and there is no life to have any meaning.

Without it there are only dead things or dying things. The dynamic force of life if dammed up and prevented from its natural expression, writhes in agony in its encasement; an encasement which is going to become its tomb and the tomb of life with it. On further reflection it occurs to me that perhaps 'joy' is not the right word. . . .

I am reminded of a tom-cat which we once kept amongst our pets when living in Fitzjohn's Avenue, London. Unlike the other animals, its comings and goings were most unpredictable; it turned up at odd moments, but only when it needed food. It used to arrive bruised and battered, with new injuries every time—torn ears, scratched face, and sometimes a damaged eye. I fancied that the catawaulings we commonly heard at night were at its instigation. Was this joy, or was it a compulsive drive, so compulsive that it ignored pain and put even self-preservation in the background? Is it joy that drives life, or is it a force that brooks no gainsaying— a force which may be joyful if we can bring it into line with our realities, external and internal, or rather if we can bring our realities into line with it, for normally and healthily it will not be denied. The force of nature will not be denied be its expression celestial, solar, tidal or biological, and we and tom-cats and leaves in the wind will be swept along by it as it sweeps through us. Ill health, mental or physical, part-death or may be only complete death itself is an effective 'cure'. Denials, suppressions and repressions, and particularly substitutions, are all part of our attempted 'adjustment' in spite of the internal stresses or agonies which we consequently endure, become accustomed to enduring, and perhaps mistake for life.

All this sublimated, purposeful endeavour, which so occupied me consciously during these years, was no more than substitutive and an attempted compensation, a compensation for that which I was endeavouring to deny, nursing like most people the idea that denial was essential in order to get on with my reality adjustments, my ego purpose. We are accustomed to encounter such endeavours in our clinical work when the formal pattern, which this drive has been forced into through inheritance or opposition, is difficult or impossible to adjust to the social structure or to reality, for instance when its form tends to be homosexual or perverted, and the ego will not permit it. There is less excuse for those who, like myself, have no endogenous excuse but who are merely the victims of a generally established conspiracy of civilisation and of economics to deny to the young, normal expression of themselves. The strength of repressive forces can be enormous, far-reaching and deep-reaching, almost incredibly so in some instances.

I once had a man patient in the middle twenties who was brought to me by his mother on account of various phobias, particularly a train phobia. This young man at first sight presented the incredible picture of almost total sexlessness. On taking his case history, there was little or no evidence of the sexual instinct, even in the familiar sublimated forms of social-sexual activity. He had no girl friend or companionship, yet he was not homosexual, but far more incredible than this was the evidence that repression had extended even to physiological function; not only had he never practised any onanistic activity, but nature herself appeared to have given him up as a bad job, or almost so. Nocturnal emissions could hardly be remembered, he had certainly not had one for over six months, and yet he was psychologically suffering from nothing more than anxiety neurosis and phobia. I mention this as, of course, one commonly sees even more complete absence of sexuality, even physiologically, in psychoses and near-psychoses. In women it is frequently accompanied by total amenorrhoea (absence of menses), for instance in cases of anorexia nervosa, but I must say in a psychologically almost-normal man such total suppression of even the physiological functions gave me food for thought.

The problem might arise regarding the psychopathology of this: whether it was due to a deficiency of the instinct, or to an exceptional power of the forces of repression. Therapeutic results seemed to indicate that in this case at least it was entirely due to the latter. Within a few months, in spite of his agonising state of tension, he was actually able to enjoy the pleasure of dancing with unknown ladies at a plais-de-danse. The theory that his trouble was due to extreme repression rather than to an absence or weakness of the normal instinct was confirmed by the fact that to start with at such dances he immediately experienced involuntary tumescence and ejaculation. This did not distress him as much as one would have expected. However, it was gratifying to note that improvement rapidly set in and extended to all departments of his psychological and physiological functioning. I think it is within the realms of possibility that he will eventually not even suffer from ejaculatio praecox. This particular disorder is infinitely more common than is usually recognised. In our civilisation, there are not only a disproportionate number of frigid, or orgastically frigid, married women (the estimate of thirty-three and one third per cent. in this country has been questioned as an understatement), but there are most certainly a disproportionate number of husbands who exhibit every degree of undesirable rapidity, thus establishing, as it were, a vicious circle regarding the symptoms of the two sexes.

To return to our problem in its more normal aspects, in so far as normality is able to survive, we might perhaps define normality as the power on the part of the instinct to survive and break through in spite of the enormous burdens and barriers heaped upon it. I had a patient once who dreamt that everybody in the world was carrying an enormous pair of castrating scissors, and columns of such terrifying apparitions appeared, led by members of the legal profession in wigs and gowns!

It is chiefly a mass of clinical experiences such as these which led me to the further reflections that perhaps joy in connection with the sexual drive behind life might hardly be the right word. I am not at all sure that it was the right word in my own particular case, certainly not in the earliest years, but I have no doubt whatsoever that it was the real drive that gave life its force, its point and its meaning, even though this meaning I struggled to disguise from myself in various asexual or antisexual forms and endeavours. The drive to integrate one's student activities had obviously to be thought of as the acquisition of learning, successful competition with one's colleagues, and the achievement of outstanding success . . . or at any rate of success.

There is no doubt that a drive there had to be, or else life would just be a matter of messing about aimlessly. Lincoln said that one can fool some of the people all the time, and all the people some of the time, but not all the people all the time. Similarly, we cannot all fool ourselves all the time, and instincts of normal intensity will and must break through the relatively flimsy untruths which we endeavour to preserve. My compensating, self-appraising pose as a coming intellectual Messiah, so valuable to me in school days, was destined to be rudely exploded, perhaps fortunately, by the uprush at puberty and adolescence of forces that would brook no denial, at least no intra-psychic denial, however successful temporarily might be the barrier imposed between these drives and environmental reality. No doubt I was not the only young man who, from inner experience, was convinced that he had a force or devil within him stronger than that which had ever been experienced by any other human being in the history of man! There was no mistaking the nature of the force either in my case.

The attraction towards a certain type or types of young woman was so compelling, so overwhelming, that it took the strongest imaginable counter-forces, such as fear, especially fear of the force itself and what it would do to me, to hold it within bounds. In its intensity, its wild, almost uncontrollable excitement, specifically in the actual presence of a young woman, I can liken it only to the force that drives certain psychopathic individuals into serious trouble, despite their sense of reality, or exposes them like our tom-cat, to the hazards of death. Fortunately for me, it was never in any real danger of breaking through control, especially physiologically. Perhaps one should, under the circumstances, thank one's inheritance for this good fortune. On a more superficial plane, its chief deterrent in regard to reality adjustments in my early days was my most devoted attachment to my mother. I am sure it is parental attachment in both sexes that is commonly one of the most effective civilising deterrents.

Of course, what is needed at this stage of one's life, and the sooner after the eruption of this stage the better, is an appropriate mate, appropriate psychologically, physiologically and materially. Only by such a means can this compelling drive of life obtain an adjustment that causes it to be a joy instead of a danger or an agony. Some experience of the stress and pain and perhaps agony of this pre-nuptial stage of life is so commonplace, is so wide and general in the experience of all individuals, that the release from it, from this tragic, unnatural situation has become the theme of practically all pleasure-reading, stage entertainment and everything else which individuals enjoy. It may be called the universal tragedy, or near-tragedy, with a happy ending. All the toils, strains and troubles, physical, such as childbirth, and material, such as economic struggle, are rightly counted at nought beside the intolerable, stressful, illness-producing deprivation of which we all have quite a long enough experience. Who can deny, under these circumstances and innumerable others, that the circumstantial evidence is complete, that the real drive in all life is the sexual urge, other instincts not having encountered comparable opposition and frustration, not at least in civilisation.

Nevertheless, we do not apparently find it necessary to impress these truths upon adolescents and young people. Instead, we offer them any and every substitution, any and every 'fob-off', as one of my patients characterised his parental and scholastic training. Well, I am afraid that as an undergraduate I was as stupid as the rest of them. I eagerly endeavoured to put every ounce of my enthusiasm into the 'fob-off' and struggled to master the mysteries of natural science, anatomy and physiology which my mentors presented to me as the appropriate direction for my life's drive. In the meantime, one lived very uncomfortably in the same sort of way as students live in these present times, either alone or with a colleague of the same sex, in dingy quarters, in bed-sitting rooms, with meals at cheap cafés or as provided by the landlady. But still one had one's ego-drive, the mastery of one's books and subjects, and one's recreational diversions, chiefly in the form of physical struggles—rugger, soccer, hockey, etc.—with one's contemporaries. What an enormous premium is placed upon the acquisition of homosexuality by life in our public schools and universities. For a young man who grows a little heterosexually mature 'before his time' this sort of life becomes increasingly unnatural and uncomfortable, and most painfully so if his instinct is strong enough to intrude itself and to keep intruding itself in spite of all his endeavours to bolster up or 'fob-off'. Something, many things, sometimes disastrous things, are constantly knocking at the door, and periodically liable to force an entry. What can be done? Very little except by himself.

CHAPTER IV

WINIFRED IN WALES

I FIRST met Winifred in a seaside hotel in Barmouth in North Wales. She was seventeen. Mr. Amery, whom I had known at St. Leonard's when I was doing that correspondence course for the London Matric., had persuaded me to accompany him on holiday as he was bent on courting his elder cousin and felt that I would serve to remove the encumbrance of her young sister. He baited me by describing her as the loveliest girl in the world. She was. Well, some might have said that she was a bit too ripe and sensuous looking for seventeen, with her cherubic lips and cheeks, wide blue eyes and generous curves, but they would not have believed what they said.

Naturally, this should have heralded the most passionate and romantic love affair of my life. It did not. Adolescent ideals, on her part largely in the form of religion, lay solidly as a defensive barrier across the path of overt passion. Love came, and for a time at least it grew, clothed in the extraordinarily beautiful garments of idealism and religion, and disguised, if not stifled, in their ethereal covering.

Of course, I had had minor precursors dating back even to childhood. I can still remember the little girl of eight years who played in a surburban London street with a group of us children, when I was barely nine. Her auburn ringlets hung about her face. Something occurred which made us decide quite openly and publicly to be sweethearts, and I sealed the bargain with a lingering kiss. There was something about the warmth and wonder of it which left me bemused for the rest of that evening, even when I was going to bed. A new wonder, a delicious wonder, had come into my life, and it was tinged with the sensuality of the softness of her lips, and some faint, warm odour of her hair and skin. However, it was soon forgotten, perhaps by the next day. At nine years of age one has other fish to fry.

At puberty, I fancy that the excitement, when observing the brown, naked bodies of young Indian girls in the sweltering heat of the plains—Umbala, Delhi, Lahore—was something of a different category; at least, it seemed to be so consciously. But certainly of the same category as that of the romantic, auburn-haired child was my reaction to the large, clean British young woman whose skating boots I laced up on the ice at Lake St. Catherine, above Lausanne, only a few years later. She figured in many dreams, but the nearest I got to her physically was from the pressure of the white-woollen-clad crowds of young people coming down in the over-packed funiculars at nights. However, the impression of these incidents and many others have left only slight traces compared to those of the outstanding puzzlement and frustration of this at nineteen years of age.

At that age, women, particularly if they were actually present, provided a background to my life of incredibly acute excitement, an excitement which ever and anon reached a degree of vivid, almost lewd intensity. There she would stand or sit, a woman or a young girl of ripening age, whatever she might be clothed in, but especially if in only a light summer frock, with her exciting body, so exciting that it evidently had to pretend to be concealed. I fancy that the concealment, or part-concealment, of clothes only added to the lure of what lay underneath. Almost indecent, this female person . . . (every inch of her was deliciously exciting) . . . as though clothes could alter the fact! Why, her aura, her femininity, percolated through any and every covering, and told all my senses that here was something, destiny, that could not much longer be deferred.

I am convinced that the excitement connected with the phantasy of the woman's body, particularly of her genital, is an hereditary memory of the sensation experienced during actual coitus, a sensation the intensity of which is always an amazing surprise when coitus is re-experienced. Phantasy reactivates the excitement of coitus in abstract, the actual presence of the female should, and normally does, intensify it by making the anticipation of it, however unconscious, nearer and therefore more real and vivid. Interest in the opposite sex is a displacement of the inherited and repressed memory of the intense sensations that our ancestors experienced in actual coitus. Perhaps all this is precisely what we mean, what we imply, when we use the term 'instinct'. Instinct is the repressed or unactivated *pattern* of ancestral experiences awaiting the opportunity of re-stimulation and release,

release from suspended and repressed tension. Everything *associated* with the forgotten past, even odours, stimulates the engram (the laid-down patterns in the nerve-tissue), the inherited 'conditioned reflexes', which we term instincts.

Perhaps the affects which I experienced were achieved only at the expense of discounting the uncomfortable and probably frustrating fact that women, or at least the particular woman of the moment, had any mind or mental apparatus of her own. It would be so much more convenient if her wonderful, deliciously seductive body and its functions were co-ordinated only by a nervous system that ensured merely the proper functioning of its reflexes, particularly of the reflex actions that would respond appropriately to my stimulations!

This is not to say that I was then, or at any time in my life, incapable of understanding the marriage of true minds ('Let me not to the marriage of true minds admit impediments . . .'). I could and can fully appreciate that what one marries, or what one should probably in every instance marry, is the mind of the chosen woman or man. It is more natural and normal and desirable than marrying a body, because after all a body, like a lock of hair, is only a fetish. (The unrecognised prevalence of fetishism in life is a subject to which I shall return. It is large enough to be responsible for the maintenance of most of the shops in Regent Street and Oxford Street, for example.) Why, all my counter transferences to patients have been to their minds. The body may have its initial, fetishistic, shop-window effect, but the mind comes in insiduously, and increasingly develops. But the mind-transference too can be sudden. Even at a wedding, I have seen an ungainly, ugly-looking bride and then something, the way she laughed and threw her bouquet into the air, has given me a glimpse of her nature and character, and I have understood the bridegroom's choice, and known that I could have married her myself.

However, the truth is I was not, at least not at that stage of my life, nor for some time afterwards, looking for a mind to marry. A body I needed (oh, how badly!) but not a mind. The fact is that the mind-need, consciously and chiefly unconsciously, was already abundantly supplied. I was already, and perhaps permanently, completely married to my beloved mother, notwithstanding her six-thousand-mile distance from me. Let no one scoff at love of mother, or even at mother fixation. It has as many social advantages as disadvantages. It is the bed-rock upon which everything in our life, everything that is us, is built. In any case, it is inevitable in the child who is going to value being alive at all, and who is going to grow up to value living. Love breeds love, just as indifference breeds indifference, and dislike breeds dislike; aggression breeds not only aggression but also fear and hate (jurists please note), and if there is one thing more than another that I can be absolutely sure of as a result of clinical experience, it is that every person spends his life repeating, acting out, the identical emotional patterns created in him during his babyhood, infancy and childhood, chiefly under the influence of his mother's feeling for him and treatment of him.

Mother's tender care of her infant is rewarded not only by his attachment to her, but by the creation of a tender, loving disposition in him, and even if it is unconsciously directed chiefly towards her, it is potentially available for transference to others. Were it not for her, created by her, it would not have come into existence at all. A wife usually reaps the harvest of love (or hate) which mother has sown.

So I had my mother, whether I knew it or not, and was not looking for another mental union. The mental marriage was pretty complete; what was left entirely out of court was, of course, the body, and I did need a body . . . not necessarily urgently, for I had grown accustomed not only to the want, but also to the frustration. On account of frustration being the regular order of life, we are hardly aware of the enormous strain and stress which we are continuously enduring and which, besides developing our powers of endurance, are often responsible for our ills, mental and physical.

Now the intensity of the yearning for this body, a yearning stimulated afresh or over-stimulated by the presence of a female body, however clothed, by its form, its grace, its movements, its speech (even on the radio), its aroma, its scent, its breath, and more fetishistically by any and every article suggestive of it: hair, comb, ornament, blouse, skirt, gloves, underwear, stocking, or high-heeled shoe . . . the intensity of the yearning for this body was psychologically nothing more or less than the repressed Oedipus need for the long overdue consummation of the marriage to the ever-beloved mother. A bodiless mother, for that is what the situation amounts to psychosexually, is an intolerable frustration. A body had to be supplied, and every feminine presence seemed to give the frustrated instinct a promise that here it was at last—the lifelong consummation about to be supplied! Anyway, here it was, literally within one's grasp.

This may give some indication of the strange restless, emotional upsurgings from within that were strong enough (only too strong) to break into, even to break through, the sublimated intellectual interests, however powerfully reinforced by ego and superego endeavour. Force met force. Instinct force met sublimated interest, and the occasions became only too frequent when instinct nearly won. At such times I would desert my gods, leave my lonely lodgings and walk . . . walk up to the lights of London and the potential excitements thereof, excitements which were, however, confined to looking, thinking and phantasying.

The reaction I can remember, on meeting Winifred, besides thinking how lovely, wonderful, delicious, was chiefly a cautionary one, that of course she was *not for me*. She was perfectly self-possessed and seemed to me very much a member of the family—mother, elder sister, and this older male cousin—who were on holiday together. But, whatever the brain or intelligence said, something deep within soon began moving stealthily and implac-ably in her direction. I do not suppose there was a breath she breathed that I did not observe, leave alone a word she spoke. It was most important to measure and take one's bearings in such an outstandingly important situation. I think there was quite an interval, several days and nights, before the over-valuation reached its zenith. This may have been partly due to the malignancy of fate, for I think it was on the day of our arrival when our party of four (we left mother behind in the hotel) went for a walk around the town that Winifred confided to somebody that she had a pain which was growing worse and that made it difficult for her to proceed. We turned back, and before long she had asked to lean on her male cousin for support, as walking was difficult. Back home, she went to bed.

That evening Francis, the cousin, said to me: 'There must be something seriously the matter, for nothing short of a total in-ability to walk alone would have led that girl to ask to lean on my shoulder.' However, the doctor was not called till the next morning. He diagnosed acute appendicitis. In those days surgical ideas were a little different. He decided that it was too late for an immediate operation, and that it had better be 'cooked' for several weeks before she was moved. (The rationale for this was that twenty-four to forty-eight hours after the beginning of inflammation, the inflammatory area, if interfered with, would be liable to infect the surrounding tissues and lead to general peritonitis. If plenty of time were given, pus would form and the poisons be effectively sealed off, thereby safeguarding the surgeon from becoming an instrument in disseminating the infection.) Thus my early contacts with this young woman were of a very unusual order. They consisted of a visit to the sick-room at mid-day, with perhaps half an hour's conversation and much looking and thinking.

Patience was at least partly rewarded, for a week later the doctor suggested she could be wheeled about in a bath chair, and it became my enviable role to wheel that bath chair daily through the shopping area and place the purchases in it, and finally to sit at the foot of it while the patient faced a lonely stretch of sea. Thus our walks and our talks became increasingly long and intimate.

In spite of the complete absence of any overt suggestion of love-making, all sorts of hidden, internal things were happening, such was the extraordinary effect, psychologically and physiologically, of the barest anticipation, however unconscious, of a release from hitherto life-long repression, of a natural relationship and natural functions. The whole world became an entirely different place; from being a potentially dull, depressing, hard and cruel world, provocative of restlessness, strife and painful endeavour, it assumed an aspect of loveliness never previously suspected. It seemed to be peopled with flowers and poetry, everything was intensely exciting and stimulating, lovely and lovable; and what is more, it was confidently felt and known that it would be so for ever. How is it that one did not know this before? How is it that one had assumed one's painful exile was all that life had to offer, that the state of exile would be as long as life itself, when, so close at hand, was available this astonishing revelation, the great surprise at the return from exile.

Analysis would tell us that the land from which we had been

exiled for so long was the land of mother, the love of desirable mother, and this experience, after age-long wanderings in a barren world, was the return to her. The conscious-level differences mattered nothing. The fundamental, emotional experience affected not only the psyche, but the heart, lungs, liver, and every gland in the body.

I believe this revival of what had for so many years been repressed never again faded completely from my life. Not the least surprising of its surprising attributes was the fact that the last thing it appeared to be, at least at this stage, was sexual. Maybe what had been found was the most effective antidote to sexuality.

Parents often, and sometimes rightly, express misgivings or alarm at the prospect of their children reaching puberty or adolescence in a co-educational school. Surely one would think in the light of the memory of one's own puberty and adolescence, that a boy and girl will get together, and there is no telling how serious a disaster may ensue. Well, boys and girls of that age do get together, and nine times out of ten what do they treat each other to? To idealism, romanticism, poetry, and maybe even love, though not so commonly as one might expect. The antidote to sexuality is certainly more liable to characterise their relationship than sexuality itself. Sexuality would seem to be a prerogative or consequence of the early homosexual relationship that comes about when the sexes are segregated, or a result of the *exclusion* of the opportunity for this heterosexual sort of relationship. Perhaps it is this very segregation, and anxiety-driven attempts on the part of us adults to protect the young from nature, that is itself responsible for the accumulation of repressed forces that are liable to initiate the very danger that is feared. Perhaps this anxiety-driven caution is the only cause of any danger at all.

I was in the throes of adolescent idealisation and romanticism. It was such an effective counter to the dislikeable aspects of the world—gloom, depression, loneliness, strain and effort—that surely I would cling to this for the rest of my days and never let it go, even at the sacrifice of intelligence or reason. It may have been the need to cling to this treasure, this new-found wonder, rather than the fear of the potential drive within, that kept the relationship on such an unspoken, idyllic level. There was something situated, perhaps between the unconscious mind and the conscious, that stood implacably between the potentially ravenous instinct and this lovely girl.

What was I safeguarding or protecting? Whatever it was, I was evidently prepared to protect it, not only with the sacrifice, or repression, of the strongest instinct within me, but even at the sacrifice of my very life; perhaps both these amount to the same thing. Analysis would reveal that this was the operation of an early *'complex'* connected with the protection of mother against one's repressed infantile impulses. (The first relationship to the mother being oral, gratification at the second oral or cannibalistic stage of development must result in one's enjoyment being coupled with her destruction.) Something takes place in the developing infantile mind designed at a slightly later stage to protect 'mother' from extermination by one's early lusts.

It so comes about that the struggle to adjust primitive instincts to the changing, socialising and integrating condition of the progress of the human race, results in many morbid by-products and illnesses. Perhaps this is an inevitable accompaniment of the biological nature of evolution. Death and disintegration are evidently intimately related to life and growth. So long as the majority survive, we may say that nature's purpose is being accomplished; at any rate, nations appear to have no hesitation at throwing any number of their young people into the cauldron of war on the assumption that national survival is more important than any sacrifice. So one wonders whether these psychological mechanisms that cheat the body for so many years of its physiological and biological needs may be the lesser of two or more evils, even if they do indirectly cause some of us to suffer mental strains, physical diseases, and even death.

The two weeks, for which I had budgeted at the hotel, came to an end, and so did my holiday money. I could not afford to continue, and yet my heart could not leave Winifred. In discussing my predicament with groups of the younger hotel guests, somebody capped all the humorous suggestions with: 'Why don't you go and live in a bathing machine?' This was greeted with roars of laughter. The next morning I interviewed the bathing machine attendant. In those days the machines were huge affairs on enormous wheels. They were dragged backwards and forwards with the tides to preserve the modesty of the bather. Five shillings a week was the rent for a machine, and I got the man to take mine a few hundred yards up on the shingle away from the hotel. I sent to my landlady in London for equipment, and within a few days I had paid my final hotel bill and moved into my new residence. Of course, it was the joke of the place. People predicted it would not last more than a week. It lasted six weeks, possibly the most delightful six weeks of my life. Not only Winifred, but practically the entire hotel, accepted my invitations to tea, and brought their own cups, etc. with the proprietor's permission. I slept in the machine, had a dip in the sea in the early morning, cooked my own breakfast, and spent most of the rest of the day with Winifred. It cost me only a pound or so a week. At the end of six weeks she, still not allowed to walk, was taken to London for the operation. Thinking the joy of life had something to do with the holiday situation, I remained, intending to return to London when the good news would tell me her illness was over.

I can still remember my feelings on that first morning when I awoke with the realisation that she was far away in London, and I was alone in this remote seaside town. I sat and puzzled, wondering what on earth I was doing there. It was obviously a completely empty place. For the life of me I could not think of any reason why anybody lived in it, and most certainly there was no point whatsoever in my being in the place. As for flowers and poetry, that could only have been a ridiculous, pathetic dream, if even that. I could not stay, I was restless beyond endurance, I, who had been so completely happy and at rest for these eight weeks, almost the entire long vacation.

If anything could bring home to a person the essential, stimulating, life-giving drive or purpose of life, an experience such as this should do so, but we are so stupid and our memories are so short. Sitting alone on the steps of that bathing machine, looking out to sea, I hardly wanted to take the trouble to find the next meal. How could one have lived all these years of one's life something like this? No organism can live without its mate; it might as well commit suicide, for it is already on the way to death. There is no growth in life beyond one generation without reproduction. Whether we know it or not, every normal man is looking for the woman, and every normal woman is looking for the man. It is at the worst the hope and anticipation that keeps us from depression and demise, whether we know it or not. These are surely biological facts. The psychological antecedents of such demise are a feeling of loneliness, a sense of the pointlessness of life, and finally a deepening depression. Friends of the same sex are not enough, should never be enough, for the really heterosexual person. With or without them, unless he has been overtaken by depression, he is restless; he is restless because he is inhibiting his impulse to find his mate. He must find love and sex, or nothing will do. I do not think my analytical mind is wrong, or that I am being fanciful, when I see this motive in many directions where it has not been seen popularly, in spite of the fact that the appropriate emotions are popularly *felt*. For instance, when I hear a popular and delightfully 'idish' song, the chief motif of which is 'Looking for Henry Lee', whatever the context or story, I detect 'Henry Lee' as a symbol for the woman's mating need. The joy in the song is that she is in process of finding him, wherever he may be hiding. In fact, she tells us so by little whoops of emotional excitement! Analytical insight should not kill the joy of anything, so long as we remember that the joy is even more important than the insight; the insight is nothing more than intelligence catching up on the otherwise blind but all-important living force.

To return to my devastating loneliness when my companion had departed, it was not long before I decided, like all of us have long-since unconsciously decided, that any form of activity, even in the wrong direction, is better than none, to conceal the fruitless meaninglessness of a situation. I packed my haversack, and that day I did the longest walk that I have ever done in my life. It was thirty-two miles, and it included walking to the top of Snowdon, and down again. I had hardly intended that it should be so long, but I think I spent from nine p.m. to eleven p.m. looking for a place to sleep in. The next day I returned to my bathing machine, packed everything, and without delay took train for London.

On arrival, my first action was to visit a florist's, a thing I had never done before in my life. I selected the biggest and most beautiful bunch of flowers that my money would run to. Perhaps it was some over-emphasis on the purity of my lady that led me to a preference for arum lilies . . . or could it . . . ? no it could not have been paranormal cognition or any sort of prognostication or omen. It was only weeks later that I recalled the struggle on the

D

face of Winifred's mother to conceal her amusement as she led me with my bouquet into the private ward at the hospital.

Winifred was sitting up in bed, looking at me silent and wide-eyed.

It was my first declaration of love.

CHAPTER V

WINIFRED IN HAMPSTEAD

THIS situation led in due course to my being invited by Winifred's mother to her house in Hampstead Garden Suburb as a paying guest. I needed no pressure. Apart from everything else, I had grown tired of my year-long residence in what amounted to a quiet slum, occupying a bedroom with a colleague who had, at the close of my first year, asked me to dig in with him, sharing a common sitting-room or study. He was a very studious man, and spent every evening with all the books spread out on the dining-room table, drawing anatomical diagrams when he was not swotting physiology. I appreciated his good example, and worked as hard as he did on occasions, but usually never for more than two or three evenings at a time. I was too restless. The second or third evening I would walk out after the meal, which we had on our return from the medical school, and visit a theatre or sit at a restaurant in the West End, with or without some gay companion.

Winifred's was a gay household, consisting not only of the widowed mother and her two daughters, but also of a third older and very much more sophisticated daughter whose betrothed, an almost middle-aged man of the world, was also a frequent visitor. There was gay chattering at the dinner table, and a generally social atmosphere not very conducive to study. I had not been there long before a young Spanish colleague of mine, the most popular and active man in our year at the medical school, full of character, bounce and energy, having visited me for a meal, pressed stongly to be allowed to join the house-party. I felt certain misgivings, but Mrs. Foster extended her welcome, and thus it was not long before there were two of us students as paying guests in her house. The evenings became a matter of piano-playings and sing-songs, whether we joined in or not, as friends frequently visited, and most of them seemed to be musical in a minor way. It was on account of the impossibility of studying anywhere in the house under these circumstances that Romero and I organised an extraordinary programme. We arranged to go to

51

bed at nine-thirty p.m., soon after the sing-songs had got under way, and to arise with thermos flask and sandwiches at five a.m. to do three hours study before leaving for the medical school at nine. This arrangement worked quite well for a whole summer and winter, so much so that we both obtained distinctions at our intermediate examinations in anatomy and physiology.

Love and Winifred were relegated to the week-ends, particularly Sundays, or a portion of Sundays, for, as I had been warned, though I had taken no notice of the warning, she was intensely religious and insisted upon attending both services at the high church, St. Jude, on the hill. Perhaps it was not surprising that even religion became for me something rather thrilling, lovely and poetical in the aura of her devotion to it.

This led to a very strange psychological situation. Long before this, as early as the age of fourteen when at that school in Simla, having learnt some science outside my curriculum and having embraced the evolutionary doctrine of Darwin, I had renounced religion as a figment of the imagination. To some extent, though probably limited, I must even have preached or disseminated my 'original convictions', for I can still remember the cold shudder that ran down my back when at this age, fourteen, one of the senior prefects bent over me while we were watching a hockey match, and whispered in my ear the awful word: 'Atheist.' I think my pang of fear was due to some anticipated persecution.

Years later at Thomas's my beliefs had become more organised, and I was better able to defend them in the light not only of Darwinism, but also of my philosophical readings, particularly those of Herbert Spencer. Nevertheless, I was a very quiet, introverted youth, and it took some years of association with religious colleagues, including Romero, who was a devout Roman Catholic, for them to come round to sharing my convictions. Maybe the scientific education which we were receiving had something to do with the changing beliefs.

And now, here was I, a 'pioneer' of atheism since the age of fourteen, finding a new inspiration, poetry and happiness in the world around me, and this long-since discarded religious belief was being presented to me as an essential ingredient of the wonder of the universe. Winifred was most anxious to convert me, and I became most anxious to be converted. I promised to try my best, and the promise included the imposition of saying some solitary prayer every morning and every night. I tried it. No doubt the most effective converting mechanism was that the arguments and persuasions came from her own lips. I listened attentively to it all, and my emotional bias in favour of conversion was very considerable. There is nothing so persuasive as love. On occasions we both felt that I was making some headway, but the tragedy of it was that I had only to accompany her to a church service to experience the ritual, to listen to the hymns and psalms, and especially to the sermon, and I would emerge more convinced of my atheistic beliefs than ever before, and the whole battle for faith would have to begin all over again.

In the meantime, personal association with me, and her developing maturity, in spite of, or perhaps aided by, protracted but friendly discussions, was leading her to some more than friendly approaches and affectionate demonstrations. We would sit very close together, and in due course the natural sequel of kissing and embracing became a part of our Sunday evening contact. I think I was more a passive and puzzled recipient of her demonstrations of affection than an instigator of these intimate situations. This now seems to me most extraordinary, but I think I must have been somewhat puzzled and wondering, though of course ecstatically delighted. Something within me told me it was not for me, atheist as I was, to thrust my own desires and compulsions into this wondrously beautiful picture. Naturally, I was very far from having any objection to her thrusting hers. It may be that my diffidence and passivity gave her courage to come out more boldly with her own impulses and desires. I think the chief deterrent for me was my realisation that *any* overt sexual activity would be incongruous with her saintly, religious emotions and beliefs.

However, without the slightest overt sexuality, the physiological nature of herself, more than of myself, clearly led to disturbances and even involuntary reliefs. Before this stage of our relationship had been long established, what I had been dumbly and dimly anticipating and what was therefore contributing to my diffidence, occurred. She suddenly began to get very acute conflict about the whole matter. 'We must not get so close together,' would I help her not to, and so on. Of course, I neither helped nor hindered one way or the other. Nevertheless, conflict grew; the poor girl evidently needed God's help more and more. I watched all this happening quite helplessly.

Eventually she found that my influence, physical and atheistic, was too much of a strain for her single-handed battle. The Church of England vicar also was insufficient help. Although she did not dismiss me—after all, I had been careful to give her no excuse for dismissal—it came about that she experienced a great religious conversion in favour of Roman Catholicism. Conversion and the priest made her radiantly happy once more. I do not remember, however, that it made her less emotionally demontrative. It did cause a renewal of her endeavours to convert me, this time to Roman Catholicism. I waited upon the priest, or Father, two or three times a week for an hour's-long instruction. But, of course, no amount of instruction can lead to faith or belief at a mature age, and my occasional sincere question so troubled the elderly man that he also finally decided that I was too difficult for him, and passed me on to a monseigneur at the cathedral. I found this theologian, for that is what he was, quite impossible, and almost immediately threw up every attempt to embrace christianity. I had tried for some eighteen months.

What had not occurred to me, incredible as it may seem, particularly in the early days of my relationship with Winifred, was to propose marriage. I still cannot quite understand why this was. I suppose we are brought up by our parents with the idea that we belong to them, and that contact with a person outside the family, however delightful it may be, remains, as it were, something outside. So many things have to be considered before one even thinks of making a real, drastic final change in one's reality, as distinct from one's emotional, situation. Besides, I had every rationalisation or excuse. For one thing, although now nearly twenty-one, I was only a student, still dependent upon my father for everything; and, in spite of the emotional conversion and pretty complete sympathy between us, the intellectual marriage, the sharing of beliefs, seemed as far off as ever, or even further. All my efforts, studies and religious experiences had reinforced and confirmed my atheism in a way that nothing else had succeeded in doing. At the same time Winifred had become, I think as a result of the pressure of her sexual conflict, more and more devotedly religious.

At the age of twenty, I was not conversant with the psychology of religious fervour, but I fancy some silent misgivings, possibly connected with a vaguely intuitive or subconscious suspicion of these matters, caused me to be more than wary of emotional approach to Winifred, and kept any such question as that of marriage practically out of consciousness. Probably I was aware of just a puzzled wonder at the phenomena I was encountering both in her and in myself. I have a theory that all living creatures are dumbly confused and wondering; in some dim way they appreciate that the phenomena they observe, understand and can cope with comprise a very small or negligible proportion of the forces existing around them, of which they have little or no cognizance. Probably they, and we, have not lost all the wisdom we pretend to have lost. We retain some in the form of wonder and a recognition of our ignorance, and an appreciation of our overwhelming incapacities, while we try to delude ourselves into a would-be compensatory confidence. The conceptual aspects of religion are no doubt very helpful to us in support of this desired compensation.

More specifically to the matter in hand, I have the theory that Winifred's struggle to enlist religious devotion on the side of her moral resistance to powerful physiological needs was, or became, an increasingly losing battle, but a battle which psychologically she could not afford to recognise as a losing one. Instead, she suffered physically and physiologically, so that insidious deterioration of health began at long last to show itself. No doubt a great deal more of such deterioration, with similar factors behind it, exists and is perhaps recognised as illness, without anybody having a clue regarding the essential causative factors.

For my own part, I fancy that this love affair, despite its enchantment and its delights, produced or emphasised certain movements in my own psychological make-up, conscious and unconscious. I may have come to the conclusion that the enchantment, the enthusiasm that spread itself over every aspect of life, the happiness and the joy, were too precious to lose. They were clearly related to some physiological, as well as psychological, awakening of otherwise repressed or inhibited impulses, desires and drives. At the same time, I may have despaired of forming a union on the intellectual plane with the sort of person, with any person, whose physical form and beauty were capable of so inspiring and enriching my life. I may even have come to the conclusion that perhaps it were better not to know her on that (intellectual) level because such knowledge might only run the risk of debunking, or at least detracting from, the heaven-sent joy which she could otherwise inspire. We are all prone to sacrifice something in order to preserve a sufficiently valuable illusion. Provided one did not form too close a conscious, or critical, intellectual contact with the inspiring personality, paradise was easily available.

When we look at a beautiful landscape, a lovely picture, or hear an enchanting piece of music, we are satisfied to feel pleasure; we do not rush to question its rational qualities or evaluate its intelligence! This affair may have pre-disposed me similarly to prefer feminine charm and beauty as something that enchanted me above everything else in the world, and not to hope for, or to wish for, an intellectual equality at the same time. This may be a poor adjustment to the reality aspects of a human relationship, but there it is. It may throw a little light on the nature and truth of the allegation that many men prefer women without brains, or even on the absurd wishful allegation by some men that women have no brains. What does one want with their brains anyway, unless of course one is looking for an employee, or a colleague, or a partner in business—or a boss to lead one? A repressed instinct is looking for something (or somebody) to release it so that the experience of tension-reduction may be enjoyed. There is much, very much, to suggest that pleasure, happiness are essentially nothing more or less than the experiencing of tension-reduction. Of course, tension has got to be there, has got to be accumulated in the first place before it can be reduced; and so the complete process consists of two parts: one, accumulation and retention, leading to the building up of a state of tension (this is identical with Havelock Ellis's concept of 'tumescence'—he has been said to have divided the whole of the life processes into 'tumescence' and detumescence!); and two, the process of reduction, release of the accumulated tension. This latter is accompanied by a sense of relief, pleasure, instinct-gratification. The phenomenon of sexual gratification is, of course, typical of this two-phase process, as Havelock Ellis has emphasised. The second phase is called by him detumescence, but more usually it is known as orgasm.

Though all this may sound absurdly technical and unimportant, to my mind it covers the widest possible field, namely that of releasing life itself, with all its accompanying enthusiasm and drive, from an all too common state of suspended animation, with its proclivities for depression, racial extinction (or, I would say, specie extinction), illness, and even death. Perhaps I was not the only young man who would gradually have withered up and died had he been placed in a womanless world, which was presumably identified with a loveless world. The source of these normal, emotional patterns undoubtedly stems from the original mother-infant situation. The tensions of increasing hunger and their periodic relief, though an early prototype, may not be the earliest. The breathing in of air (oxidation) neutralises the chemical state of impending asphyxiation and relieves its rising tension. The basis of the happiness of living is as fundamental, as *chemical*, as this. Can you do without it? Try!

Despite all these truths about myself, and reflections upon others which I have been recording, I should add that the release of alloerotic libido from repression, so happily brought about by this first love affair, though it caused a period of wonderment and a need for new considerations, never entirely beguiled me into thinking that it would be a complete susbtitute for an enquiry into the nature of myself and of things and people around me. It did undoubtedly draw my attention to the fact that I had been leaving something out of my book, perhaps the most fundamental, important, essential thing. We have to eat in order to live, but that eating should be a complete answer to all our needs in life is hardly the same thing; nevertheless, without eating no other needs would arise. I had learnt that one has to love and to be loved in order that life should be worth living, but it did not follow that the drive or need to understand what we were doing and what it was all about, the nature of the macrocosm and the microcosm, was thereby rendered superfluous.

The reality fact of primary importance in my life was still that I was a student at St. Thomas's Hospital Medical School, now in my third year, and with the need to complete my mastery of anatomy, physiology and pathology before passing on to clinical work in the hospital. Emotional development associated with this love affair had undoubtedly given new zest to my activities and enthusiasms in every direction. The story of those student days from first to last is a story, not of lighthearted, youthful adventures, pranks and gaieties, but a story of absorption, occasionally, though only very occasionally, breathtaking absorption in the wonder of the universe as revealed by the study of physics, chemistry, biology, and the more specialised attention to anatomy and physiology. Absorption in these genuine revelations was more than an escape from the anxieties of the enforced extraversion inseparable from the close association of large numbers of young men of my own age. To me, it had long been the very book of God, a new and worth-while God. How could the world continue with the criminal activity of teaching children in school and everywhere the alle-gorical, legendary 'explanation' of the origin of the world and of ourselves, when here were detailed, accurate, unquestionably factual matters, showing the very mechanisms of this amazing and wondrous aspect of reality.

For instance, did everybody know, were all children taught, that living matter began and developed under the salt water of the early seas? Did they know that every form of plant life that grew on the land outside the sea had originated as nothing more than a parasitic growth, arising from the more fundamental under-water plant life; a growth which had, from its submerged source, reached the air and, still a parasite, developed chlorophyll with which to utilise the ingredients of the air? Did they know that every form of terrestrial animal, most interestingly ourselves, had emerged out of these prehistoric seas, and that they, one and all, carried within their body-substances the identical salt and mineral concen-trations which originally existed within those seas? Did they know that the egg, human or otherwise, should be regarded as practically identical with the original unicellular marine animalcule, and what is more, that it still carried, as it were, its own pond, albeit a salt-water pond, around it in the form of the fluid in which alone it could live and develop?

Did not all this biblical teaching amount to an incredibly stupid denial of this invaluably stimulating, exciting and mind-developing, real knowledge which extended far deeper than the realms of bio-logical science, right down, I was even then sure, to the very elements and their locked-up energies themselves, without break in the developmental and evolutionary process?

The knowledge of which I, together with most adolescents

even of to-day, was humorously, though not tragically, innocent was that the first essential for survival, a matter which in practice superseded all these interesting matters of philosophy, was that one had sooner or later to become primarily absorbed in the economic struggle, that the world of man was so constructed that this economic struggle was liable to take precedence in urgency and importance over all these deeper and more absorbing matters. Perhaps that is why so large a proportion of people in the world remain ignorant or insufficiently appreciative of these things, and arrest their intellectual potentialities with the acceptance of the outworn, legendary philosophies and theories of over two thousand years ago. Another matter, of which until later I had been more or less innocent, was that the inherited nature of man, of myself, unlike his conscious preoccupations, was designed or evolved by nature to ensure the perpetuation of the species, and thereby to maintain for ever a breaking-point load upon his economic struggle. These truths are in due course so forcibly borne home to us that I have, in my more mature years, found myself telling enthusiastic, intellectually idealistic adolescents that they would not really begin to know anything until they had per-force to support themselves, and not properly even then until they found that they had to support not only themselves, but a growing and multiplying family.

These reflections at the moment remind me of an incident that happened in Bombay several years later, when I was a Medical Officer in the R.A.M.C. during the first world war. A colleague and I, having bought large, thick, port-hole glasses from a merchant in the bazaars, and having ground them into lenses, or rather optical mirrors, had constructed what was at that time the largest telescope in India. We were being, perhaps sarcastically, lionised by a group of our elders and betters at a dinner party, given in our honour, and probably being looked upon as a couple of interesting curiosities or crazy youngsters. An older man, baiting me, asked what I proposed to do with my astronomical researches after the conclusion of hostilities. I rose to the bait, and smugly replied that I intended to extend my survey of the heavens to include spectro-scopic photography and an analysis of the chemical consistency of the celestial luminous bodies. Probably by that time he had enough of me. His remark burnt into my mind, never to be forgotten. He said: 'By the time you are forty, you will think yourself lucky if you can manage to keep yourself in cigars and whisky, and that is about as much as you will care for spectroscopic photography.' My attitude at that time, spoken or not, was that if maturity meant such intellectual degeneracy, then the sooner one drank oneself to death the better. However, I can now see that there was a lot of realistic wisdom in his banter.

If whisky and cigars were still left out of my calculations, the reality of other gratification needs, which I had much earlier ignored, had been brought home to me by the advent of the love affair which I have been recording. The reason for recording it is just this: It gave me vivid evidence that there were more things in heaven and earth than were, or had been, dreamed of in my philosophy, and what is the good of a philosophy if any matters, leave alone big, overwhelming matters, are left out of its account. These things serve to remind us, philosophers or not, that the essential bases of life must be recognised, accepted and catered for before it is healthy to devote one's energies (perhaps only surplus energies are available) to the further-sighted, not-so-immediately essential considerations and requirements. What were those headaches which so impeded Herbert Spencer's work that he could only dictate to his secretary for very short periods, ten minutes or so, without having to interspace his mental activities with bursts of violent exercise, such as rowing round the lake when they were sitting in a rowing boat, until he felt ready for another bout of dictation? Perhaps if we read his extraordinarily condensed and complicated paragraphs we can better answer this question! But more seriously, I am inclined to think that, like many intellectuals, he had for too long been endeavouring to concentrate on philosophical thought at the expense of natural needs. The basic instincts have a way of coming back symptomatically on those who would ignore their demands.

The experience of my love affair told me, in a way that no other lesson could have told me, that trying to be a Diogenes before one's time, however natural the intellectual enthusiasm may be, is apt to lead to symptoms of introversion, loneliness and depression, symptoms which are prone to inhibit or undermine the very source of the energy and vitality which one wishes to use intellectually. I suppose many students get over this difficulty, in part at least, by their recreational sporting activities, but to my mind these are based unconsciously upon more or less repressed homosexual potentialities. I could never find the thrill in rugger, cricket, or camping in the Officers Training Corps, which some of my perhaps more fortunate brethren seemed to feel was enough to give life its punch and enthusiasm. The advent of the relationship to Winifred did for me what everything else had failed to do, in spite of its physical frustrations and the enormous amount of food for thought, puzzlement and insight which it provided. As I have indicated, the biologically induced enthusiasm and excitements gradually tended to become increasingly inhibited by the mental incompatibility of philosophical and religious beliefs. For her, no doubt the immediate emotional satisfaction accruing from religion, both from its beliefs and its practices, including its music and singing, was far greater and stronger than that of the painful, frustrating pursuit of scientific and philosophical knowledge. Maybe this religious satisfaction was necessary for her health, at least in the absence of, or under the circumstances of the inadequacy of, biological gratification. I was tough enough to do without religion; in my case, it seemed my critical desire for truth gave me no alternative, but I had seen that I was not tough enough to defy nature's primary demands indefinitely without losing the joy and enthusiasm of life itself. As it turned out, neither was she.

The most heartbreaking development in the first quarter of my life was that during my absence abroad, both before and after qualification, occasioned by the war and Army medical service, Winifred's health began to deteriorate. Perhaps I had robbed her of even the anticipation of consummating our love relationship, for my puzzlement at the incompatibility of our beliefs had held me back from any overt promise or anticipation of our getting married. I may have wondered whether or not it were understood. What she wondered I do not know. The general impression is that our enthusiasm for each other had begun to fade. Perhaps the separation owing to the war gave us more time for reflection and hastened the cooling of the relationship. From the news I periodically received, I gathered that she was tending to become more and more devoutly religious. There had even been the familiar, perhaps not-to-be-taken-too-seriously (she was, after all, no more than twenty) talk of her entering a religious order as a novice. Whether

her deterioration of health was directly psychogenic, or whether it was indirectly due to the frequent long periods of fasting that she adopted, I think with the unconscious motive of reducing sexual feeling, I do not know. I had been away little more than a year when, after a brief period of wasting, she was found to have contracted tuberculosis.

In the light of more recent clinical, psychological experience, it seems to me significant that this previously very healthy looking young woman should not only contract tuberculosis, of which there was no hereditary diathesis, but that the disease should actually have started, as I was informed after her first surgical operation, in the ovaries themselves. A life of medical experiences still inclines me to believe that organic disease, like all other ills from which we suffer, like all our behaviour and activities, originates within the psyche (often phylogenetically), probably in unconscious conflict, and is commonly first revealed by the individual's reactions to his social environment. I was learning such lessons, even at that time, and the intensity of the distressing emotions consequent upon this awful news, and what I then felt to be my unbelievably cruel and irremediable loss, only served to impress the lesson more deeply and irradicably upon my mind.

However, real grief, like melancholia, is silent and deathly. Mine could not have been so real, or if it were, it did not remain so real indefinitely. At some later date I produced a spate of sorrowful and rather morbid verse. Perhaps I fancied myself as a great bereaved lover and poet. But in actual practice I proceeded to go on with my life as though nothing had happened. Nevertheless, I imagine that, as probably occurs with every bereavement, my mind periodically reverted to the feeling of a ghastly sense of loss, though eventually at increasingly long intervals.

CHAPTER VI

MEDICAL SCHOOL

IT takes the amateur in astronomy to be constantly impressed with the overwhelming nature of the magnitude of the universe and the incredible measurements of interstellar space. The professional is far too busy getting on with his practical mathematical calculations. The study of astronomy may serve to console us with constant reminders of the insignificance of human life and tragedy. It may even become almost a sort of 'schizophrenia' on its own account! My recollection tells me that I was not so completely 'schizophrenic' as to be indifferent to the general, social or public interest which, with the other one or two members of our scientific group, I was arousing, particularly at the time when we installed the great telescope on the roof of the War Hospital in Bombay. Naturally one liked to think that the rest of the world was being somewhat schizophrenic in confining its thoughts and interests to the very limited sphere of terrestrial human activities, and actually seeming to ignore this incomparably greater and more important cosmos.

If we were not schizophrenic enough to confine our attention to our immediate physical and gratification needs, limiting our foresight to economic requirements within our limited span of life, we might, in attempting to bear in mind the longer and wider view, find that we had lost ourselves emotionally in a limitless waste, and pre-disposed ourselves to a more morbid and dangerous schizophrenia!

However, it seems that I was not destined to devote my life to this wide field of research and enquiry. Perhaps it was not the aspect of the universe which I found most difficult and most puzzling. Adler has it that it is specifically his weakness which a man signals out for his attention, for attempts at compensation or over-compensation. My weakness, the thing that puzzled me most, was the nature, specifically the mental nature, of my fellow beings, stemming, it may be, from my puzzlement about myself. Observation of them probably increased my puzzlement.

I am reminded of the story I heard about the late Professor

Spearman, the great academic psychologist. A colleague of his
once said to me: 'Spearman never could even begin to understand
psychology. He was so puzzled, so much at a loss regarding
people, why they did what they did, why they thought and behaved
as they did, that he could not rest. It was on this account that
he devoted his whole life and energy to trying to find out how
their minds worked and why. Unfortunately, he chose the wrong
method. He chose experimental psychology; he tried to measure
exactly what the central nervous system did under specific
laboratory conditions. Of course, this built up a limited structure
of knowledge, including the isolation of one or two laws, such
as his 'g' factor, but the knowledge was more physiological than
psychological, and at the best it did not seem to be at all easy
to apply outside the experimental laboratory.' He concluded
with the patronising remark: 'Poor old Spearman, he never
did understand human beings, and died just as puzzled as when
he started.'

I would, however, be more inclined to liken my own case to
that of a patient who fairly recently consulted me. He, too,
was a doctor, in fact an operating surgeon, and his analysis gave
me in retrospect some insight into what had probably been my
unconscious difficulties when starting my university life at St.
Thomas's. This man was very much more shy and introverted
than I had ever been, and this led to an easier and more vivid
discovery of the unconscious roots, not only of his withdrawal,
but of withdrawal in general. I do not wish in this light work
to go into exhaustive clinical details, although this would be
the only way of proving the conclusions at which we arrived.
This man's main symptom was that he was terribly shy and uncomfortable in the presence of any social group, particularly if it
consisted of men, or included men.

I believe that my early days at St. Thomas's Hospital, the
puzzlement I felt at suddenly finding myself amongst all these
young men, the wonder and the strain and the tendency to introversion, were all due to similar mechanisms in a minor form, which
this patient helped to reveal to me so vividly. I had suddenly
been thrust from a secluded family life in Lausanne, where I had
had only two or three occasional friends or acquaintances of my
own age and sex, with a brief interlude of perhaps three months at

a seaside resort doing a correspondence crammer course for the London Matric., into this hubbub of social activity. My life in Switzerland, altogether of nearly three years' duration, had been, for the most part, rather lonely. The private tutor is a very poor substitute for school, and had undoubtedly increased my tendency to introversion. I can remember that these hearty fellows seemed to me, or some of them seemed to me, very puzzling and a little frightening. I daresay I concealed my reactions pretty successfully, and at the most appeared only a bit quiet and taciturn. I had not made friends very quickly, had found my own lodgings, and spent the first year pretty much in solitude, apart from the actual classes and work at the medical school. It had been towards the end of this year that another student, perhaps one who was even more seriously minded regarding his studies than myself, had sought me out and suggested that we joined forces for the rest of our curriculum. Thus came about the situation which I have previously mentioned, which prevailed throughout my second year of study, and which was only broken when I preferred, shortly after the second long vacation, to remove to Winifred's house in Hampstead Garden Suburb.

I have indicated that while overtly and consciously absorbed in my professional or scientific studies, I was, subconsciously at least, as much absorbed in the puzzling effects of my reactions to my contemporaries, both male and female. My reactions to males, as I recognise now, were for the most part defensive or obstructive. The advent of the female, in the shape of Winifred, opened the new and unsuspected world of release from potential morbidity, and stimulated emotions and phantasies which had been too long repressed—all this, in spite of the difficulties which it encountered, and its failure to provide any permanent solution for this aspect of the problem of human adjustment. What funny things we are in our youth, if we do not succeed in being thoughtless, or perhaps it would be kinder to say, if we do not succeed in being absolutely normal. I am not the only one who nurses a theory that some degree of abnormality is a necessary, an essential, precursor to any advancement in human knowledge. This may be particularly, if not exclusively, true of psychological knowledge. Many are the patients who have said to me: 'Doctor, you cannot know anything about me or my psychology, you cannot possibly ever understand.

E

One has to have experienced and suffered the same things as I have suffered to be able to understand them. You are so horribly and impossibly normal!'

Only recently a publisher in a foreign country, who had not only published a translation of one of my small books but had been in the habit of writing voluminous letters of a personally analytical nature, finally arranged to pay me a visit. Under the circumstances, I invited him to dine with me in my flat. Throughout the evening I suspected that he had something on his mind, but it was not till after midnight that he finally broached the subject, and it was therefore two a.m. before he left. I wondered why he had taken so long to start, as he had surely intended to tell me this from the beginning.

Shortly after, a compatriot of his, the lady who had translated the small book in question, also visited me. In the course of the evening, she let slip a hint that I was not exactly the sort of person she had expected to find in the light of her study of my writings. It took all my powers of persuasion to get her to explain. Finally she came out with the pretty broad hint: 'Well, doctor, you seem to be much more of a business man than I had expected.' I gathered from this and some further remarks that she had thought that a person who wrote as I did would be at least every inch a dreamer, if not an actual schizophrenic. Perhaps it is possible to have more than a nodding acquaintance with the realms of the unconscious and yet be fully alive to the superficialities of the so-called real world around us. I hope so.

Nevertheless, the lady was mistaken. Business men should be warned of psychotherapy as a profession, or should we say as a trade. I met one or two in the early days who had not been warned off. The poor things have no patients at all now, and I personally am not inclined to send them any. Would you?

The principal subjects of the second medical examination, namely anatomy and physiology, are regarded as the scientific basis of the practice of surgery and medicine, and are therefore pursued, almost to the exclusion of all else, for the extraordinarily long period of two academic years. At the end of this time, one is supposed to have mastered them pretty thoroughly. One has dissected with one's own hand every inch of the human body, including the brain and the nervous system; one has pursued this physical examination into all its branches, the skeleton and bones, including a knowledge of every tubercle on them and groove in them; the microscopic appearance of all the body's tissues (under the title of histology) including sections not only of the brain, but of the spinal cord at every level, and in addition the whole of an interesting subject called human embryology, which is devoted to a study of the development of all these things within the uterus from the unicellular egg. Physiology is more concerned with the functional, chemical and physical, activities of the body and its ingredients, but it and anatomy, particularly the specialised and microscopic aspects of the latter, are to some extent complementary or supplementary to each other. It can be appreciated that by the time one has negotiated the second medical examination (second M.B., B.S.) at the end of the third year, one is or should be something of a scientist in these special departments, but is, of course, in no sense a surgeon or a physician.

I think the authorities who arrange the medical curriculum are particularly concerned to avoid the subsequent practitioner adopting unscientific methods and becoming a bit of a 'quack', and the intensity and thoroughness of these studies are insisted upon for the purpose of forestalling such an undesirable contingency. It is as though they said: 'Stick to the scientific facts of anatomy and physiology, and you can't go wrong.'

It took me a great many years, and a considerable experience of general practice, to find out that, however sound and admirable the motive for this thorough scientific grounding, if one sticks too strictly to it, though admittedly one cannot go wrong, it is only in comparatively rare instances that one can go right either! This is due to the fact that, although there is so much to learn about these sciences, they do not and cannot go far enough to link the essential (i.e. initial) causes of human ills to the physical basis of mind and body. Apart from direct physical and chemical relationships, our contact with our environment, our relationship to the external world, material, social and personal, the relationships upon which our welfare and survival depend, are all initially of a psychological nature, and each is accompanied by variations of emotional tone. There is no mental happening, emotional or otherwise, that has not its physical accompaniment. To say this is perhaps going no further than to say we know of no mental process without a physical basis (e.g. a brain). The trouble with the science of medicine, with its anatomical and physiological bases, is that our knowledge has not yet advanced far enough to link these almost imperceptible changes initiated by reactions to environment, such as social environment, with all the subsequent physiological and physical happenings in the body. Thus we have an enormous gap in our knowledge, a gap between the study of the mind and that of the body.

I am reminded of that old gag which asks the question: 'How did Mr. Baldwin get into the House of Commons?' The humorous reply is in terms of the physical (c.f. anatomical and physiological) movements of his leg muscles. The joke is most relevant in this context, but the advocates of an exact scientific basis for medicine and surgery, in terms of anatomy and physiology, have never seen it! Medicine, and even more so surgery, in so far as they are endeavouring to be exact sciences, are, as a rule, dealing exclusively with secondary products, resulting from a mental process, specifically from a mental process consequent upon some failure to adjust our environment to ourselves, or ourselves to our environment. The mind, including the intelligence, has been born and has developed solely to assist the body to overcome frustrations of the life-process, and subsequently frustrations of instinct gratification, a higher level of the same thing.

What makes the problem deeper and more difficult is the fact that failures may be cumulative from the earliest days of our life, and in my conviction can have extended to us through past generations Lamarckian-wise. To my mind, this is no more mysterious than the recognised phenomenon of the inheritance of instinct, instinct which must in turn have been acquired through environmental adjustments appropriate to that stage of evolution. *In short, we inherit both healthy and unhealthy reactions, and develop them one way and another in the course of our life.*

Now, the exhaustive study of the sciences of anatomy and physiology, and the insistence that medicine must be based exclusively upon them, limits the function and utility of the practitioner, limits his work to that of endeavouring to deal only with secondary or end-products, and tends to limit his enquiry accordingly. The result is that less scientific bodies, such as the Church, not to speak of the Welfare State, have taken it upon themselves to regard the initial and essential causes of human ills as their prerogative.

In spite of all this, when it comes to the actual practice of medicine, at least outside the precincts of a hospital, every practitioner cannot fail to recognise that the vast majority of his patients is suffering essentially, and always initially, from something which he can in no wise correlate with his scientific studies of anatomy and physiology. So true is this that it is, generally speaking, the practitioner who is more a man of the world or a person with an ordinary capacity for understanding other people's troubles who is infinitely more helpful and successful than one who is exclusively a scientist.

The undergraduate in medicine, especially up to the time of passing his second medical examination, having had no contact with sick people or troubled people, has no conception of all this. He has no reason to doubt what he has overtly and implicitly been taught, namely that to understand the scientific operation of the laws of physics, chemistry and physiology, is to be able to mend the things from which people suffer, and for which they will consult him for the rest of his life and theirs. A terrible shock is in store for him. The more scientific and serious he has been, probably the greater will be his subsequent disappointment. Generally speaking, he receives no warning of this.

This is the sort of position that I and my colleagues of the same year were in when we happily negotiated our examinations in anatomy and physiology, and excitedly anticipated being launched into the actual practising departments of the great hospital adjoining our medical school.

The first job one is asked to do is usually that of casualty dresser; one is a sort of unqualified assistant to the casualty officer on duty at the moment. Casualty officers, like other housemen, are of course a race apart. They have recently achieved the dizzy height of medical qualification; they are now real doctors with white coats and a stethoscope sticking out of the pocket. As qualified medical men, they have a position of some responsibility. The casualty dresser who serves under them spends his duty time mostly with dressings and bandages. He learns a subject of considerable practical importance—the different types of dressing for different conditions for instance—and with his absorption in this, may not have time to dwell upon his disappointment at finding that the actual menial work seems hardly worthy of the depth and breadth of his exhaustive scientific studies.

There are, of course, moments of special interest or excitement, such as after each casualty session, when one has a group of cases for gas and minor operations. Usually one is at first thrilled at doing real, practical work instead of mere study. One learns to hold a gas mask on a patient's face, and in due course to understand not to asphyxiate him; one learns to open whitlows, to stitch cuts, and to do a hundred and one other things which will probably comprise a considerable portion of one's active surgical work for the rest of one's days.

One is not taught to take much notice of the people or the personalities that carry these minor troubles—cuts, burns, whitlows, carbuncles, etc.—on their persons into the Casualty Department. One is too busy, and in any case it would not usually be very relevant. Nevertheless, some of us got a smattering of the characters and natures of a large class of persons with whom we were not previously very well acquainted. At the same time, we achieved a good deal more personal contact with one another, as well as to a lesser degree with an occasional nurse. In my days at the hospital, any relationship with a nurse was as cold, official and distant as it could possibly be. Anything approaching even the slightest friendliness was more than discouraged. In consequence, I came to regard nurses simply as official automata, and was very conscious of their somewhat hostile and contemptuous attitude towards undergraduates. This was about the year 1913, but I believe that things have changed very much since those times. Perhaps the disrupting and socialising effect of two wars has had something to do with these changes.

There was a certain amount of hilarity and boyish horse-play amongst us as casualty dressers which was not so noticeable during the years when we were all studiously engaged in the dissecting room and physiological laboratories, with an eye on the coming second medical examination. It was, to some extent, an interim period of relaxation from serious studies. In many respects, I think it was a more valuable education, for it brought us into immediate contact with life in its very real aspects. From being almost pure scientists, if not merely theorists, we were now more ordinary human beings.

No doubt I had matured considerably during the three preceding years, had got the measure of my associates to some extent, and was considerably less introverted than during my first year at the medical school. I now fancy that this part of my education may in a sense have been more valuable than any other. It was more practical in preparing me for a life which was to be daily and abundant contact with my fellow beings.

My own tendency when working in hospital, particularly when I moved to the less hustling bed-work in the wards, was immediately to become more interested in the individuality of the suffering patient than in the jocular nonsense of my contemporaries. At the same time, I think I was a little gratified to notice that the great man, the visiting consultant who took us on his rounds to teach us, appeared to share this interest in the personalities and individualities and sufferings of his patients to a more marked degree than did any of the juniors, not excepting the less junior ones amongst them such as registrars, assistant physicians and assistant surgeons. I felt that perhaps like him, I too could look a little beyond the pathology of tissues to the mental state of the individual who had the disease, the suffering, and, occasionally, the anxious anticipation of death.

It was not entirely easy for me to understand why so many of my associates seemed so unfeeling and indifferent to the tragedy of human illness, and so exclusively concerned with its anatomy, chemistry and physiology, or perhaps more truthfully, so concerned with their own individual welfare in passing eventually their qualifying examinations. It was almost as though some of them said: 'What does it matter if these people live or die? What matters to me is that I pass my examinations.' There is, of course, some excuse for them in that the life or death of patients was not their personal responsibility.

I remember my first awful shock on entering a post-mortem room. It was our duty to attend the post-mortem of any patient for whom we had been medical clerk. Generally speaking, the whole firm, that is to say, the visiting physician in charge of the ward, his house physician, and his entire retinue of students were led on occasions to watch the expert post-mortem operator per-

forming his task. The post-mortem room was situated at the far
end of the medical school. The first time I walked into it (it must
have been on a Monday when the number of bodies is at least
twice as many as on other days,) I saw nine or ten stark naked
people, each stretched out on a slightly sloping table with grooves
and a gutter in it, something like a large kitchen draining-board.
The corpses included, besides a few elderly ones, several
quite young people, males and females, and two or three
children. There they lay, silently stretched out, each with a
clean post-mortem knife lying along the centre of his or her
chest.

I think poets or would-be poets should go into such a room as
I did, alone, and listen for a time to the silence. Truly, it would
tell them a great deal, and give them as much food for thought as
the happier and more pleasant aspects of life can give. I remember
afterwards saying to a very practical and materially-minded colleague of mine, that I felt that from the point of view of a relative
or friend, to see one's nearest and dearest laid out like that,
stark naked, stiff and cold in a public room, with a knife on the
chest, would be a devastating, horrifying and rage-provoking
experience. 'Would it not be better, would it not show more
respect and appreciation of the human aspects of the situation,
at least to cover the body with some sheet or gauze?' He was
indignantly opposed to my idea and sentiment, in spite of the
fact that he was a Catholic. He said emphatically: 'That would be
inviting a lot of sentimental tosh and nonsense. These are just
bodies, corpses, not individuals.' (I was inclined to think that
perhaps to him they never had been individuals, and could not
be even if he had known them as patients.) He continued with
emphasis and heat: 'This is a scientific, not a sentimental or
religious situation. To treat it as anything else is to confuse the
issue.' I was quite appreciative of what he said, and in the end
came to think he was right. Perhaps it would seem rather absurd
to perform a sort of religious honour to the corpse, and then
immediately to proceed to slit it down the middle, as one does at
every post-mortem, from chin to pubes, and extract by systematic
sweeps of the knife every bit of its contents, including even the
soft palate, fauces (with tonsils), entire tongue, pharynx, larynx,
etc. all through the vertical slit which descends from the chin,

and subsequently to lay all these things out on a large general counter for slicing and more detailed examination.

These extensive post-mortems are performed by the expert with great speed, as well as great thoroughness. I have known a man regularly to get through six, seven or eight of these in less than a couple of hours' work. The state of the post-mortem room when he left it was, of course, indescribable. It would remain for the regular attendant in his gumboots and thick rubber apron to hose it, and to stuff the scattered organs and everything anyhow into the open corpses. He would then proceed with an enormous needle and strong thin twine to stitch up the elastic skin in large rapid stitches from pubes to chin. A final hosing directed on to everything, and within a short time each body would be ready for the concealing shroud. So this was a necessary and essential aspect of medical science.

Our erstwhile landlady, a workman's wife, who had carefully looked after and fed my colleague and me in those semi-slum lodgings when we lived together during our second and part of our third year, subsequently died in St. Thomas's Hospital of a perforated gastric ulcer. Her husband came running to us both, and with great emotion told us that one of her last expressed wishes was that my colleague and I should attend her post-mortem 'in the interests of science for the benefit of humanity.' We looked at each other silently, and both knew that it was the last thing that we would do.

I mention these matters as they are undoubtedly amongst those which have to do with the formation of the character and psychology acquired by all medical men. Certain modification of the usual or ignorant attitude towards life and death must take place during years of an accumulation of such regular experiences. The average or untrained person would probably be consumed with horror at the prospect of cutting up a corpse. He is apt to forget that such wholesale cuttings up become a portion of the curriculum of every doctor in the course of his training. In addition to this, human life and death, as well as illness, are of course the doctor's very stock in trade. Similarly, he becomes familiar with the body, its structure and every detail of its functioning.

Later on, during the period of work as Casualty Officer at St.

Thomas's Hospital, I grew accustomed to giving anaesthetics in the main operating theatres under all sorts of conditions and at all times of day and night. I remember on one occasion having to sit on the anaesthetist's stool at two o'clock in the morning, hardly able to see, with operating sheets hanging all about my head from above like a tent, while I poured chloroform on to the interior of a small mask, and then held it over the mouth and nose of a man who faced downwards over me, for the surgeon was standing on some sort of steps above my head. The patient had been brought in after a road accident with a fractured skull and signs of cerebral compression due to haemorrhage in the membranes under the skull. The surgeon a jolly, though amazingly capable and outspoken, young resident, had trephined and was now using parrot-bill forceps and pulling off large chunks of bone, throwing them over his shoulder as fast as he could go. He said it made him think of the familiar operation on the breakfast egg. At the same time he was keeping up a flow of aggressive banter at the expense of the nurses around who were assisting him. 'Wake up, Nurse So-and-So. Have you been out on the tiles all night?' and so on. The troubles he got into through such excesses usually left him smiling and undaunted. My concern was to try to keep in touch with the patient's pulse as felt in his facial artery, and with his conjunctival reflexes, under these conditions so difficult for observation.

There were many such curious happenings, strange fare for one whose tendencies, unlike those of this particular surgeon, were essentially towards introversion. I have recorded this and other similar incidents throught this book to correct any possible assumption amongst the medically untutored that matters connected with life and death are necessarily harrowing to those professionally engaged in dealing with them. Emotions such as would be felt by a loved one or by a relative identifying himself with the patient, would not increase one's skill in dealing with medical and surgical exigencies. Usually the contrary would be the case. That is one, though only one, of the reasons why I deprecate very strongly the frequent practice of leaving a desperately ill person in the charge of a near relative, particularly if the latter happens to be a doctor or a nurse. The danger to the patient is exceeded only by the mental sufferings of the attendant.

On the other hand I would like to correct any impression that doctors, surgeons and nurses are necessarily heartless or cruel or indifferent to matters of life, death and suffering. It is a popular mistake, an ignorant misconception, to assume that the reaction of those in charge of a medical or surgical case must be essentially an emotional reaction, that they must feel either the pain and distress of the patient in sympathy with him, or be experiencing a sadistic indifference. The truth is that they are usually far too busy trying to help him to have time, thought or regard for their proclivity for emotional reactions of any variety. Whatever job we do, and become accustomed to doing, we learn, or should learn, automatically to disregard, or to suppress from consciousness, emotions which would interfere with our efficiency in performing it.

There was amongst us a rather manly and mature-looking foreign student who, even from the time of our second year at the medical school, when we were doing our anatomical dissecting, was for ever asking people to accompany him to one or other of the four or five operating theatres in the main hospital. He argued that it was helpful to our anatomical studies to watch the major operations being performed. I think each of us had in turn been persuaded by him, although I personally felt somewhat uneasy in the students' gallery of a theatre, feeling that I had no right to be there as I was not yet studying surgery.

Reflecting upon this man, and his addiction to this form of recreation, it has since occurred to me that he probably obtained some sadistic pleasure in watching the live, human body being carved about. What is even more probable is that none of us was immune to at least a modicum of voyeuristic gratification in seeing adults of all ages and both sexes pretty thoroughly exposed while under the anaesthetic, for instance during the moments when the sterile sheets were being placed over them prior to the operation, and again when they were being removed after the stitching. Like all such sexual interests, short of coitus and of gratification, familiarity tends to breed contempt, and in spite of my father's expressed opinion that only females should be permitted to tend females, even when it was no more than the bandaging of an ankle, (an opinion which I treated with contempt), I have, by dint of experience, come to the conclusion that this familiarity is a very good thing in that it leads to an immunity to emotionally irrelevant situations which would, to the unaccustomed person, tend to be sexually stimulating. I think this view can be extended to a generalisation exemplified by the movement from concealment, so marked in Victorian times, to the present-day relatively free exposure of the human body of both sexes. When ladies wore very long skirts, the sight of my lady's ankle was probably of a more stimulating, erotic interest to the male of those times than the appearance of a girl in a bikini would be to the male of to-day. Surely this is a movement away from morbidity, and its general implications are obvious. If we hide nature, we suggest something special or exciting which the revelation of reality dispels. I dare say to the naked communities of some parts of the world, everything is pure, or at least harmless.

Voyeurism, like all perversions, is the price we inevitably and inexorably pay for concealments and, in general, for all frustrations of instinct—painful, usually unnecessary, and certainly inadvisable in view of the price. The opposite to perversion, the negative to its positive, is neurotic symptom. They are opposite forms of reaction to instinct frustration or part-instinct frustration. One or other is inevitable, whether visible or not, whenever instinct frustration prevails. A not uncommon *form* taken by these morbid products of denial of nature is that of punishment. It reveals itself in all cultures and at all ages, under its heavy disguise, as more sadistic (i.e. more perverted) than that which it punishes.

In the same way that a doctor in the course of his training becomes familiar with the body, so he gains, though more by necessity than by training, a unique degree of intimate familiarity with the human mind, unless of course his defences in this respect are morbidly powerful. As a dog-breeder or a kennel-maid gets to know her puppies and dogs, so a doctor gets to know human beings in the physical aspects of their life, and in those mental aspects that are most fundamental and important for their healthy functioning and well-being.

I remember the great and very human founder of the Tavistock Clinic, London, Dr. Crichton-Miller, who used, when he had the power to insist that no doctor was employed there as a psychotherapist unless he had previously had experience as a general practitioner. His theory was that this 'real doctoring' was the only adequate training for the understanding of the human sufferer, particularly for the understanding of his mind, and specifically for the understanding of the distresses in it which led him to seek assistance with or without organic disorder.

CHAPTER VII

PLAY

NOT every aspect of one's student days was as serious and gloomy as those I have been describing. The youthful joy of living will fortunately break out and free itself in spite of the heapings upon it of studies, examinations, science, disease and death. I can still remember, in the medical school days, a fine, lusty young Italian with a powerful operatic baritone voice, who used to sing when walking down those interminable gloomy corridors between the old-fashioned lecture theatres. Fifty or more of us might be sitting, crowding one of the amphitheatres, listening to dry-as-dust expositions on bones or something, when we would hear the reverberating melody of this young man, singing at the top of his voice, coming closer and closer until finally the lecture had to be suspended until the opera passed on its way. Nobody ever interfered with this spontaneous exuberance.

Then there was my incredible friend, Romero. He would sit by himself in the fourth row, immediately in front of and above our physiology lecturer, who, incidentally, was a very serious and dangerous man. Romero would dust snuff, or was it pepper? (I don't know which it was—I wish I had asked him), on to his note-book, and when the lecturer turned to add to his diagram on the blackboard, would blow it skilfully towards him so that it settled around his head like a small cloud. Thereupon his serious and emphatic discourse would be interrupted by a series of violent sneezings, while the entire class tried to stifle its merriment—and fear. As Professor Mellanby turned again to the board, Romero would step noiselessly from his seat into the gangway, and bow ostentatiously, resuming his place again before being noticed, and then proceeding with the snuff game. Not the least amusing thing about this performance was that when the Professor, sensing some joke at his expense, though unable to glean what it was, let fall some criticism directed against the isolated culprit, the crazy Romero's mood changed entirely, and he lapsed into a serious and indignant state of sulks, (as though *he* were the injured party) which he did not attempt to conceal.

Such phenomena as these exhibited by the young, though evidently most enjoyable, left me at a complete loss. I could not understand how anybody could behave like this, and if I had any glimmer of understanding, it was completely dispelled by Romero's indignant reaction to the lecturer's mild and more-than-deserved criticism.

Then there was that Easter holiday at Mayleigh with its succession of ridiculous adventures: Romero's proposal of marriage (and acceptance) by two seventeen-year-olds on the same morning. Fortunately they were friends and mutual exchange of confidence forestalled heartbreaks. There were the football games on the village green; Romero serenading the shop-girls on the spokes of his upturned bicycle in the middle of the high street; Romero tap-dancing and collecting money for the barrel organ man and monkey . . . and hundreds of other spontaneous high-spirited incidents. The total absence of self-consciousness, this complete naturalness and exuberance, in spite of an audience or because of it, was a thing I envied from the bottom of my heart. I realised it was quite beyond my capacity and never ceased to marvel at it.

Probably God has been kind enough to endow every large group of students with at least one lively wit to lighten their darkness and enliven the deadliness of life. Why he wanted me, of all people, with him, I could never make out. It must have been some mother or father—transference phenomenon.

Having joined me at Winifred's house in Hampstead Garden Suburb, it was not long before he lapsed into his old habit of greeting me by seizing me by both ankles and lifting me straight up into the air. My ankles were perpetually in a bruised state. Therefore, at long last I fled, and found another residence up the road. It was more important for me to get away from him than to stay with Winifred. Romero helped to carry my things there, but before long he was suing to join me again.

However, I was not the only one who came in for his horseplay. I remember the time when Romero and Harry, both sturdy young men, were on casualty dresser, major week together. I should mention that casualty dressers during their major week had to sleep near the Casualty Department of the hospital in a two-bedded room reserved for them, as they were on duty throughout the twenty-four hours. There was a great hoo-ha through the department as nobody could find the casualty dressers who were urgently needed. I happened to be about, and a worried sister accosted me, and asked if I had seen my friends. I had not, but I joined in the search. I looked again into the bedroom which had already been investigated and declared empty, and was just about to close the door on the apparently empty room, when I observed a slight movement of one of the bedsteads. Of course, I immediately looked underneath, and there were the missing pair, locked together in an all-in wrestling embrace. They were dragged out, both too short of breath to make a sound or offer any explanation.

It was notorious in the hospital that during their duty together they were continuously in a physically exhausted state, each with bumps on his forehead and other signs of wrestlings and struggles. I have seen the fun begin. Romero, who was incredibly strong, would, out of sheer exuberance, whether or not anyone else were present, seize the Irishman Harry by his jacket and pants, lift him off his feet and throw him across the room, perhaps on to or about an easy chair or settee. Harry would rise madly to the bait, and try to gain a mastery over Romero, an impossible ambition, but he would not give up, and the result would be that Romero had perforce to continue to struggle against him until both were exhausted.

The source of such behaviour must essentially be a muscular need pressing for expression over and above the routine of mental activities. It is comparable to the play of schoolboys and puppies, and no doubt has its function in the promotion of health and growth and muscular development. In this instance, both young men were outstandingly capable scholars. Perhaps such activities kept them healthy at the same time.

Why am I recording these trivial things? Surely such behaviour is of a piece with that of infants, jumping up and down as they do, mere expressions of unorganised *id*-activity, behaviour necessary at this stage of life for the relief of id tension. Their more mature equivalents would doubtless be censored. Behaviour at instinct level, when it is sufficiently primitive or childish or unorganised, meets with no opposition in our part; we regard it as just innocent delight, are relieved and pleased to see it, and may even wish that we could take part in it. It is an expression of impulses at pre-Oedipus, pre-genital levels, innocently and harmlessly revealing themselves. They correspond to a stage of pleasure life before the

Pandora box was opened; in analytical language, to a stage before structural conflict arose in earnest between instinct gratification and parent or introjected parent (superego) prohibition, to a stage before we had to 'murder' our opposing, frustrating parents in order to gratify the genital, sexual need which was unconsciously developing in us.

It is the Oedipus complex and the social organisations, including religious ones, which develop from it and the resulting structure of society, which make it impossible for us to recognise that any sexual activity can be equally harmless and 'innocent'. Adam was no longer innocent when he had eaten the fruit. He had disobeyed the command of the Father who reserved all 'knowledge' (sexual knowledge, i.e. sexuality) as his prerogative. Thus socially, religiously, psychologically and in every way an enormous premium is placed upon infantile pre-Oedipus modes of self-expression and release of tension, 'clean fun', 'innocent' happiness.

None of these modes of release is comparable in effectiveness and efficiency to that which reaches organisation with developing maturity. Whatever manifold and multiple forms of reduction of tension living creatures enjoy, none of them is complete or completely health-giving without the addition of their equivalent sexual forms. The animals, from birds to mammals, recognise this intuitively without question or dispute, and indulge their mature functional apparatus as naturally and innocently as their pre-genital impulses and desires. It would seem that it is only man who has stigmatised maturity, restricted and confined it in obstructive rules and regulations as though it were, or were liable to become, something anti-social and destructive of one's neighbours. So much so is this the case that if an author went on to describe the expression of experiences comparable to those which I have been describing, but in the sphere of sexuality, he would be stigmatised and his works would be in danger of being regarded as pornographic, or, like me, he and readers alike would become so familiar with all these matters that they would (again like me) genuinely not want to write or read about them—at least not for idle pleasure.

All these young men and young women are not so infantile through and through, nor all the time, as my selected samples of behaviour would indicate. Nevertheless, I am inclined to believe

F

that their sexuality, like Romero's kissings of the village girls behind the bushes, can be as wholesome and harmless (even if 'innocent' is not the appropriate term) as the infant's spontaneous jumpings up and down. Why this horror of literary description of them, why this dislike of their accurate introduction into consciousness, why this stigmatisation of such attempts as pornographic? I think there are several inter-dependent aspects of an answer. The first obvious one is that accurate descriptions of sexual activities would either so seduce the reader's interest from attention to all other parts of the story, that owing to the immeasurably greater strength of the sexual impulse, everything else might become just waste of time and therefore irrelevant, or that it would arouse unduly his or her resistances so that the book would be cast aside (maybe to be picked up again surreptitiously!) What is the reason for this? Surely it must be a recognition of the fact that this omission (of sexual detail) is insisted upon because sexual behaviour is emotionally such an important matter that it would, if not omitted, take precedence over all the relatively trivial and unimportant matters which we do not censor.

The valuable contribution which I have to offer here is that I believe if there were no censorship of these matters, they would then, and then only, be seen in their proper perspective and be able to take their proper place in our minds in relation to the relatively less emotionally stimulating or disturbing incidents such as I have been describing. A further aspect of this truth may well be that if we were accustomed to reading and writing about sexual matters and sexual details without having to de-sexualise or de-emotionalise them, 'pornography' would be, or would become, impossible. There would be no need and no tendency to perverted accentuation of this or that aspect of the truth, even of the emotional truth. I think our minds would be enriched and that it would be altogether a happier and healthier world . . . and a more 'innocent' one. Hate would be less; surely it is engendered as well as aggravated by the frustrations of censorship. I do not suppose we are in any real danger, in fact I think we would be in less danger, of tearing one another to pieces, any more than we were really in any danger of murdering the father or mother during our Oedipus stage of emotional development. Must we perpetuate the nonsensical

Oedipus conflict by our lives, our religions, our writings and our readings, in our social organisations, in our censorship, and most important of all, in our liberty of thought by deforming restrictions placed upon our very minds? I am confident that this has much to do, perhaps everything to do, with our international, social, mental and even physical ills—yes, I will say it: not excluding war as a psychic phenomenon and cancer as a physical one—at least by fostering a predisposition to them.

It would seem that half our emotional life, the most overwhelmingly important half, *and for that very reason*, has to be left out of our conscious thoughts, descriptions and writings. If it were not so, might it not become as commonplace as the equivalent of the infant's jumpings up and down which I have been describing?

Before leaving this discussion of the innocent high spirits of adolescents I must say that the not necessarily less innocent sexual interests and activities of adolescents, have a healthy and necessary place in nature. Perhaps it is only when their vigour is sufficiently healthy, and their drive sufficiently determined to overcome the enormous and seemingly insurmountable obstacles placed in their path by a world united against them, that subsequent health in life can be assured, or subsequent morbidity averted.

I am referring more especially to the very widespread psychosexual morbidities that we encounter in our professional work, which are so frequently the determining factors not only of much depression, inhibition, or a state of half life only too common in civilised countries, but also of so large a proportion of definite illness, mental, nervous and organic. It has been shown by more than one author that when, in the course of an organism's growth and development, a highly organised instinct ripens to maturity if at that point the instinct is prevented from exercising its functions and is successfully inhibited or frustrated, it may never again succeed in expressing itself or functioning. No amount of tuition, education or encouragement can recreate that which has been, as it were, nipped in the bud.

Perhaps if we stopped a child from jumping about and using its legs as it felt inclined, and then at a later or more adult stage of life wanted to recreate the muscular potency of its legs, it would be found that the opportunity for healthy movement having been lost, such healthy movement could not be regained. This par-

ticular experiment has never been tried deliberately, at least not
for sufficiently long a time to prove it in this form, but there are
analogous experiments in the realm of animal psychology and
functioning which have been tried. For example, the following is
suggestive: A kitten, at a very early stage of its development,
will instinctively catch mice, kill them and eat them. If now at a
point when it is just ready to do this, it is consistently prevented
from exercising this instinct, it will, when it grows up to be a cat,
be unable to kill mice, and no amount of encouragement or training will be able to restore that which has been prevented or
destroyed. It can never be taught to kill mice.

Thus, we see in our clinical laboratory—the consulting room
or analytical session—men and women who are incapable of
responding normally or appropriately even to such a very fundamental and primitive instinct as sexuality, specifically to the act
of coitus. What has happened to them during the equivalent
kitten stage? Very often it is nothing more or less than that upon
which civilisation has appeared to them to insist. They have
swallowed these apparently conventional teachings hook, line and
sinker. Some of these unfortunate people are diligently occupied
in now trying to remedy the defect Usually their first attempt in
this direction is to read books on the subject. I have elsewhere,
I think, told the story of the wife suffering from acute anxiety
neurosis who at first, in answer to the question, asserted that
everything was normal between herself and her husband, and who
subsequently, through associations to a dream in which she experienced revulsion, terror and horror (comparable to her phobia)
at the approach of a bird 'if its wings touched me, I think I would
scream'), confessed that that was identical with her reaction
when her husband approached her sexually. She went on to explain:
'You see, doctor, he tries very hard. He does it all out of a book,
I know it all so well now that I could almost name the page of the
book he has in mind at the moment, and then of course it never does
any good; it is all over with him almost before it has started. I
cannot bear it, I feel I shall scream. It is driving me crazy.'

The truth is that the man was psychosexually impotent, but he
was doing his best to get his ego to do service for the instinct whose
functioning he has lost at some earlier stage of his development.
Admittedly this may have been long before adolescence, but it

is quite likely that the premium placed on asexuality throughout adolescence and after had not helped.

At St. Thomas's Hospital I did not learn the true psychopathology of such conditions and of their more advanced and more morbid consequences and sequelae, in spite of the fact that our teacher in psychiatry, the late Dr. Stoddart, knew them all very well. My chief recollection of this delightful and most likeable gentleman is of his demonstrations of mental cases, conducted at Bethlem Royal Hospital, where he was the Medical Superintendent. In those days Bethlem was situated in Lambeth; the premises have now been transferred to Monks Orchard, and the old building is, I believe, used as a museum. In the large hall at Bethlem, packed with an unnecessarily large number of students who had practically one and all come for the entertainment value of the demonstrations, Stoddart would present his selected cases, and so far as possible, get them to do their stuff. I can still remember a fascinating young woman who appeared in an exotic silk shirt-blouse and a pair of white flannel trousers, one leg of which was deliberately rolled up to just below her knee. She talked all the time in an extraordinarily excited and vivacious manner. I can remember that her talk, tumbling over itself as it did, was quite delightful, if rather disjointed. Stoddart explained that he had let her, for this occasion, dress as she pleased in order to help to demonstrate, amongst other things, the manic tendency in choice of clothes. This was more startling in those days than it would be now. Perhaps all the world, or the youthful elements of it at least, have moved in this generation more in the direction of mania than of depression, to judge by the choice of clothes.

It was some years later, when going the rounds of Bethlem, that I met this lady again, then having her second manic attack. The sister opened the door of a padded cell, only to slam it hurriedly and to call two or three nurses. She explained: 'That is the third time to-day that Freda has stripped off every stitch of her clothing. We will have to put her in one of those canvas overalls that she cannot strip off or tear.'

Knowing the hypersensitivity of the skin during some phases of mania, and the intolerance of some sufferers to the sensation of clothing, I tried as tactfully as possible to hint to the sister that, after all, the weather was very warm, perhaps warmer in the padded cell, and did she think it likely that the patient would catch a cold (maniacs never do) if, under the circumstances, she were allowed to have what was apparently her wish, and be naked. Of course, I might as well have been advocating free love to an Archbishop of Canterbury.

In my opinion, mental nurses should all have psychoanalysis before being given the custody of mentally ill people. I have heard it said by a very prominent psychoanalyst, and how truthfully, that it can be guaranteed that an unanalysed person will treat anybody suffering from nervous or mental trouble incorrectly. I am inclined to extend this aphorism and to say that it can be guaranteed that an unanalysed person will treat a baby, infant child, adolescent, or for that matter adult, incorrectly. Perhaps it would not be too much to go on to say that even analysed persons, however well analysed, are also bound, at least on occasions, to treat all people, ill or well, young or old, incorrectly, and this, not only in relation to the depth and excellence of their analysis, but particularly in relation to the state of their digestion, for every person, however well analysed, is still human and therefore subject to the physiological basis of emotional reaction.

For this reason and for others, possibly none of us can expect complete security or uninterrupted immunity from the hazards of fate. I am inclined to think that probably the best safeguard, the best assurance of correct treatment, is nothing more or less than that which it has always been, before our psychology was dreamed of, namely love. The mother who loves her child will, under all ordinary or average circumstances, treat it correctly enough for it to grow up as good as she is, if no better, and itself as capable of love. Personally, I doubt whether any science or scientific training, analytical or otherwise, can really take the place of healthy, normal, unmorbid love in its therapeutic value and effects, whether the thing we are dealing with is infant or patient.

However, love, like everything else in the world, even if we are agreed that it is the best that one human being can offer another, still has its pitfalls. The mother's love for her infant, needing her as it does to feed it, whether she be wolf or lady, is the one thing that ensures its survival, and more than this, through the ingraining of the same emotional reaction, ensures that when that infant becomes a mother, it will similarly love and succour its progeny. Thus, the mother's love ensures more than the survival of the infant, even the survival of the species in the image of its parents. What then are its pitfalls?

The pitfalls of love are secondary to morbid situations otherwise induced. For instance, if the human female behaved in accordance with nature's design, she would probably have an infant yearly, would transfer her motherly love, or the greater part of it, to the last comer, and the others would naturally grow away from her and escape in accordance with their developing maturity and nature's plan, just as fledglings leave the nest and fly away, perhaps never to see their parents again. But, owing to the complicated economic structure of our society and possibly other factors, we interfere with nature's plan, with the result that the human mother frequently has no later arrivals, or insufficient of them, or too widely placed, for a natural reduction of the intensity of her love for her growing infant to diminish appropriately to its increasing age and lessening need for her and her attention.

This mother-love is all the more likely to reach injurious proportions if, as so frequently happens in our civilisation, her relationship to her husband has lost some of its initial fire, and particularly, of course, if it has cooled down to such a degree that her love-needs in life are essentially transferred to her child or children. I am sure this is, to a large extent, what happened in my particular case. It is common enough. Under these circumstances the mother, especially when there are no subsequent children, is driven by the inherited instincts and emotions within her to cling to her growing child with her love, for she would be lost without this relationship necessary for her health in the absence of a more natural and desirable state of affairs. Such a natural and desirable state of affairs would be a continuation of passionate love with her mate and a regular succession of babies. Economics in this cultural world forbids. It may be that the morbid emotional states which result in consequence of our sense of economic reality, in short our sense of reality, will eventually cause more suffering, ill health and risk of extinction, than if the reality were ignored in favour of an 'insane' acquiescence to emotional pressure. It may be that around us there is already some evidence to be found for the truth of this seemingly crazy statement. Does not history show that the lower classes, who take relatively no heed of their economics and realities, but produce large families without regard to their sustenance, periodically overthrow the 'far-seeing' aristocracy who have put security and economic security before a blind subservience to the 'instinct of propagation'? And have we not had recently, with the news of the linking of China and Russia, some evidence that nations backward enough to behave on an instinctual, emotional and non-reality level, may threaten to swamp, perhaps to swamp out of existence, more cultured peoples who have on the whole been more reality-minded in limiting their multiplication in accordance with the food and amenities available.

In short, until we, with our precious reason, came upon the scene, nature worked in accordance with old-established laws, the psychological representatives of which were instinct and emotional pressure. Now, our developing reality sense has found something better. Perhaps it thinks it can, like Canute, stem the tide of nature's age-long forces. Maybe it would be better for us to acknowledge them and adapt ourselves to them. We may, by our efforts, improve upon the speed at which the tide is carrying us in its direction, but if we think it is our job to go the other way, against the tide, can we be sure of any progress whatsoever, or might we be more correct in anticipating merely exhaustion and demise?

I am recording these reflections, which to some may seem unnecessarily banal, but I think the fact is that a very large proportion of thinking people have not recognised these banalities. To my mind, for instance, religious teaching throughout the world is largely an exhortation to exorcise the forces of nature, often represented as the devil.

During his analysis, I exercised what influence I could, short of entirely spoiling all progress, to restrain an angry and aggressive patient from 'knocking the block off' his immediate boss in his office. The strain of suppressing his impulse did not prove too much for his control. He never did knock the senior gentleman's block off, but he did suffer from such a degree of increasing tension and strain that he found in the end he could no longer tolerate going on with his job. He handed in his resignation. Ever since then, this patient has argued that if only I, his analyst, had not been so stupid as to prevent him from following his natural drive and knocking the boss's block off, all would have gone well. He would have knocked it off, and thereby drawn the attention of the directors etc. to the horribleness of this man and the undesirability of employing him in the office. This boss would have been sacked for ever, my patient's tension relieved, and he, my patient, would be still happily engaged pursuing his office vocation. Well, well . . . whether this is so or not, a consideration of an abundance of such material, certainly some of it far more convincing, suggests to those who are daily hearing evidence of the forces in the human mind that a substitution of powerful emotional drives by reason is not immediately practicable. At present it belongs to the dreams of idealists. In the meantime there are wars, and there are badly brought up people who, through the psychology of their master's badnesses, bring about wars. Nevertheless, they should not prevent us from trying and hoping that our developing reason will help us to modify the expression of our loves and hates in accordance with the demands of reality.

No doubt the psychological phenomena, with which I am here concerning myself, are all nothing more or less than manifestations of the growing-pains of humanity, or, to express it more accurately, the pains of the evolutionary development of humanity from beast to man, from instinct-driven animal based upon the age-old voice of nature, through the experience and adjustment thereof towards the new emerging animal, the one that has an increasing reality sense and a developing reason. Possibly amongst our common mistakes is the one of thinking that we can jump suddenly from the one state to the next. Growth and progress, like the movement of the incoming tide, is never smooth. It goes in *little* jumps, backwards and forwards, and in the course of our mental and psychological evolution, many curious conflicts and morbid situations arise. The stresses, discomforts and illnesses we suffer, mental, physical, individual, national and international, may, like neurotic symptoms, be based on nothing less than the structural conflict between id and ego, id being the old-established order of instinct gratification (pleasure principle) and ego being the latest development of the reality-sense-tendency to impose modifications upon it. Viewed in this, probably correct, light our sufferings may be regarded as inseparable from the evolutionary process, or just a later stage of the early 'struggle' of animate matter against inanimate.

CHAPTER VIII

1914

AFTER I had been working for a little over two years in the wards of St. Thomas's Hospital, my father arrived on holiday from India. I had found him a boarding house in Adelaide Road, Hampstead, and as the long vacation was due at about the same time, my brother, five and a half years my junior, and myself were expected to devote our time to sharing his holiday.

He was amazed to find how little we knew about the great city in which we lived, and set himself the pleasant task of showing us all its hidden mysteries, historical buildings, familiar-to-him city restaurants, and so on. His conduct on these jaunts was painfully embarrassing to me, and only less so to my brother. He was hail-fellow-well-met with everybody, and talked in a loud voice, even in the midst of crowds. For example, in the underground lifts, which commonly held anything up to fifty silent city clerks and other Londoners, he would continue his conversations, personal or otherwise, oblivious to the fact that everybody could hear, and was not averse to getting them all to join in, particularly the lift attendant, and other railway officials. Everyone seemed to enjoy it and take it good-humouredly, except myself and my brother.

Perhaps I had never forgiven my father for his utter failure to understand me when I was a boy. An apparently introverted or dreamy infant and child may well justify misgivings in a parent's mind. I believe, but I cannot remember, that my poor, misguided father had even had resort to the inestimable crime of trying to 'wake me up' by an occasional slap on the head. According to my mother, she soon put a stop to the development of this tendency on his part. Have you ever slapped a cub in the presence of the tigress! However, I can well believe that even a single atrocity of this sort could produce traumatic effects. Try as he might, father could not begin to understand or to appreciate the dangerous anachronism of the un-boy-like boy. I have heard that he was much relieved and, in the end, positively excited, though bewildered, at my school and examination reports.

At the time of this London visit my father was in his early
fifties, and his social character was a mixture of that of the cos-
mopolitan and the confirmed colonial. Throughout his life he had
been a wanderer; he had worked in every capital in Europe and
learnt nine languages. His travels and various occupations had
taken him to the Middle East, the Far East, Canada, and especially
the United States of America. He had no inhibitions in regard to
the over-quiet and reserved London crowds. He was always well-
dressed, laughing and debonair. Walking through a city street one
morning we passed a woman sweeping the pavement in front of
her shop. He promptly stopped, told her that she was holding her
broom the wrong way, took it out of her hand and proceeded
to demonstrate by doing the job for her. A little crowd of passers-
by collected. My brother and I edged away, trying to pretend we
did not know him. However he took no notice, and finally handed
the broom back to the smiling woman, insisting that she held it
in the way he showed her.

Then there were the interminable operas to which he took us,
usually in the less expensive seats. The one type of show that
was beyond me in those days was opera, but my father himself
commonly grew impatient, and after the first act we would leave,
go to a saloon bar for him to have a drink or two, and then very
often go to another opera for the rest of the evening. He had mixed
with every creed and type of society all over the world, told me
he had dug the roads in Paris as a young man, and was particularly
sympathetic and friendly towards the working classes, with whom
he evidently felt a great comradeship. It occurs to me now that his
social, emotional reaction to all people was that of the cosmo-
politan to the parochial, and this applied also to his wife and family.
I never understood him. I fancy that I might now do so, but it is
of course too late.

It was while I and my younger brother were on a walking
holiday with him in France that the first world war became
imminent. We were just able to get back to England before the
Prime Minister announced the declaration of war against Germany.
In spite of the hospital's opposition, many of us students succeeded
in getting our names put down, particularly at the Admiralty,
for temporary service as Surgeon Probationers or some such
medical or surgical work as assistants to qualified officers.

It was not long before my turn came round and, together with three colleagues, I was assigned to a hospital ship called the *Sicilia*, which was carrying a shipful of wounded Indian soldiers to no other place than Bombay, where my parents and sister resided. My father had returned there, at the end of his holiday, to resume his job of superintending mills. As I had not seen my mother for some five years, although we were still the most devoted couple on earth, the prospect had its compensations. We spent the greater part of our time putting hot fomentations on septic wounds. Most of the soldiers cried like babies whenever their wounds were dressed. Every would-be conqueror and warmonger should have a compulsory course of service doctoring. I can think of no more curative experience.

The I.M.S. officers, with whom we messed, were an extraordinary study. They were almost one and all full of high spirits and low stories. At this latter accomplishment however, the somewhat blasé young purser of the ship excelled anybody I have ever met before or since. Anything and everything that was said, even a hiccough, reminded him of a little gem. Even in those days, it was of passing scientific interest to me that these educated people, once their scholastic ambitions had died out and they were segregated from female company, made their chief topic of conversation, and apparently the chief source of pleasure and hilarity, funny stories all of which, without exception, had sexual implications. Was sexuality as important as this? Admittedly the chief tendency in these jokes was to burlesque, satirise or debunk any valuation placed upon it. Yet what was the psychology of this exclusive preoccupation in life? Evidently one factor was to compensate for the absence of wives and sweethearts and women in general, but essentially it was, I rightly thought, itself an attenuated and socialised form of sexuality, a form that went down rather better with plenty of whisky and soda. Try as I might, I could not care for it very heartily. Yet I would have contemptuously repudiated any allegation of being a prude. Probably my unconscious homosexual component was still too much repressed.

I had for so long been cooped up in the scholastic world that the voyage and reunification with my family had particular interest for me. I was crestfallen when a telegram arrived from the War Office that we, Surgeon Probationers or 'dressers', were to be brought back to London to resume our studies and get qualified as soon as possible.

The fairly sudden change from the warm climate that we had been in to the cold of the English Channel and Southampton Water on a February morning did curious things to us. Many of the students got a malarial attack, and I got one of the worst attacks of neuralgia I have ever had. This had something to do with a subsequent flogging of the theory that my neuralgia was malarial in origin, but this, like every successive theory of its causation, had eventually to be discarded, and one had to accept the un-welcome fact that there was nothing that could be found to account for it. In the light of my psychoanalysis, some fifteen years later, I came to the conclusion that it was psychogenic, and intimately connected with the strength of my determination to strive after an ascetic, asexual life which was inappropriate to my inherited nature. I did not strive after this for its own sake so much, but as a necessary condition of scholarship.

So I thought in those days. I had not been analysed, and was still able to get away with my rationalisations, having no con-ception that asexuality stems from unconscious phantasies of castration. Castration anxiety is the only force strong enough to stop sexuality, and it is bound up with the Oedipus Complex. But shall we for the time being stick to our superficial motivations. I think that the strain of enforced extraversion put a greater burden upon me and aggravated my condition of restrained and controlled tension (feminine-component defences) which had developed into one of my main characteristics. I was of the intro-verted, thinking and studious type, and circumstances were not permitting me to enjoy the amount of solitude necessary for my health. Therefore I shall not pretend, as I tried to do to others, that adventure and continuous sociability were an exciting, happy or congenial state of affairs.

After a few months of revision work at St. Thomas's Hospital, I found myself sitting for the first qualifying examination, the M.R.C.S., L.R.C.P. All the usual competitive and scholarship examinations in medicine and surgery, which were normally held in one's last year before qualification, had been waived on account of the war, and thus one did not have the opportunity of any pro-fessional honours. Naturally, the programme was to get legally qualified as soon as possible in order to serve one's country in a really useful capacity.

I negotiated both parts of this qualifying examination, held consecutively, and, with a few friends, annoyed the hospital authorities by immediately getting ourselves bundled into military uniform. The hospital was trying to insist that every one of its students who qualified should do at least six months of a junior house job before being taken away by the War Office. They rightly held that the work of St. Thomas's was just as important as running around in a field ambulance, and they could not carry on very well if they had no junior staff. On this account, my colleague Harry and I compromised, and were given the curious title of Honorary Temporary Lieutenant, R.A.M.C., while we were officially lent by the War Office to St. Thomas's to do three months Casualty Officer and Resident Anaesthetist. One advantage of being in uniform was that we were no longer liable to be presented with the white feather that certain ignorant women were at that time regarding it their national duty to hand out to young men not in uniform.

In the casualty theatre we would often do a dozen or more operations in a morning, including such things as extracting hidden needles, under X-ray guidance, from hands and buttocks (what difficult messes some of those jobs were!), joyfully dissecting out little tumours, such as cysts, occasional circumcisions, and chiefly the removal of tonsils and adenoids in children and infants. For T's and A's (Tonsils and Adenoids) the children were brought in by the nurse already dressed in waterproof cape and waterproof tight-fitting cap, so that there would be no blood on their hair or clothes. Children thus dressed were automatically regarded by the operator as listed for the removal of tonsils and adenoids, were immediately anaesthetised, and the operation rapidly performed. Now, my mind is literally agonised at the thought of the psychological traumata that we, and those like us, must have been inflicting and are still inflicting on the poor unprepared children; but in those days I was too ignorant . . . or was I? . . . no, I think the appreciation of the 'crime' was deliberately suppressed for the sake of expediency and peace of mind.

Not the least of the educative effects of medical or surgical practice is its tendency to test the capacity one has for confidence in oneself, and to develop the germ of any self-confidence which is there. In these respects, at least, I do not think I was lacking. What adolescent is? Can it be a virtue as well as a fault? Perhaps I was reaching an age when I was beginning to feel that I understood everything, including even people. I may have become over-confident, or at least given some such impression. I remember the occasion some years later in the war when I was second Medical Officer on a troopship sailing from Bombay to Basra, in Mesopotamia. I had become very studious again, and was busy reading the works of Haeckel, much to the annoyance of my senior colleague, who had been a medical missionary. We dined at the Captain's table, and one of the ships' officers, decrying the learning of our profession, was saying: 'What would you do without practical people like us? If we were not on the ship, you would never be able to navigate it and to get it to Basra.' The Captain chipped in with: 'Don't you believe it! If we all jumped overboard, Berg here wouldn't turn a hair. He would take the ship anywhere, right into any bleeding harbour.' That man did not like me, although I was a most studious, inoffensive person, and had given him absolutely no cause for any hostility, so far as I knew. It may be that my contributions to the conversation had stimulated some inferiority feelings in him, for I heard at Basra that he had almost publicly declared that he would never sail with me on his ship again. Shortly after this, an order was given for him to sail back from Basra with a load of troops, and, as ill luck would have it, for me to be the Medical Officer in charge. The dispensary key had been lost, and the drugs had to be checked by the Medical Officer before embarkation. This quite senior Captain was in a ridiculous state of anxiety. He even took chisel and hammer himself, and broke open the dispensary door so that I would have no grounds for official complaint against him. He seemed to be convinced that I was after his blood, heaven knows why, for such ideas would have been more foreign, I think, to me than to anyone on earth. He was a nice, simple fellow, almost old enough to be my father, and I quite liked him, but nothing would alter his conviction.

This was not the only instance I encountered, and still encounter, in my life of the paranoid tendency in normal people. It is incredibly widespread. Maybe we are none of us quite immune from it, perhaps every person we meet is more or less prone to groundless suspicions, unnecessary defences and unreasonable hostilities. Those in whom these proclivities are at all marked, and we encounter many in every walk of life, are more psychological strain to those around them than is generally appreciated. They prevent our relaxation and naturalness, for we have everlastingly to be on the alert lest we offend or hurt them, tread on their corns or stimulate their paranoid suspicions. They never have any insight, and are totally unaware of the strain and trouble they cause. The result is as though one were dealing with, sometimes even living with, mental patients, and must for ever have an eye on their reactions so as not to provoke their paranoid symptom. What a relief it is when one is with people who are relatively immune from this tendency!

The essence of most novels, stories, dramas, as well as the awful happenings of real life, is the varying paranoid tendencies of people, commonly identified with the concept 'character'. It is the 'character' (or paranoia) which provides the essence of the peculiarities in the phenomena of human relationships. It is a very deep-seated and pretty well incurable disease. The psychoanalytical theory is that paranoia is founded on repressed homosexuality. One may conclude, in keeping also with Jung, that every male has a feminine component which is repressed and of which he is usually totally unconscious, and that every female has a masculine component. My own, perhaps rather vague, clinical impression is that any powerful repression of such an essential force as the sexual instinct pre-disposes the individual to paranoia or to paranoid tendencies and reactions. Freud's view is in keeping with this, as it is usual for a homosexual proclivity to be more firmly repressed than a heterosexual one, but I feel I have evidence of paranoid *tendencies* at least that have their source in repressed sexuality of the heterosexual as well as of the homosexual variety. One might expect that nobody can repress absolutely from consciousness a component of such a strong instinct as the sexual without there being the possibility that its energy, being so strong, will be liable, under certain circumstances, to break through repression in some altered form. This is a classical mechanism, particularly in regard to the pre-genital component instincts, in the formation of every psychogenic symptom. To my mind, paranoia is just one of the symptoms or one of the forms, which

G

these repressed forces, whatever their unconscious nature, can take. It is a form that touches the very highest reasoning functions of the mind. I believe that nobody's reason is quite untouched by these forces. Character, or character-formation, is just one of the symptoms, or processes, formed, like all symptoms, out of the repressed and repressing forces which serve to use up, or to *bind*, the energy of the unconscious conflict. When it is manifestly paranoid, such as in established cases of paranoia, it shows more clearly, I think, that the individual's sexuality is being used, exercised and bound in this very remote, complicated and curious way.

I think now of a young graduate from one of our older universities, who consulted me a few years ago. He was, like a lot of paranoiacs, hardly ready at first introduction to give me his tremendous confidence. He first needed his suspicions removed regarding me, and how I might use the information if he divulged it. By dint of great patience, sympathy, and perhaps pretending to be as stupid as he was, the first hints tentatively emerged. He wanted to know what I thought of a certain remark that one colleague in the laboratory where he worked had made to another. The remark seemed to me a transparently innocent one; for instance, it may have been some question as to what sort of weather the other man thought they were going to have for the week-end, but having encountered such cases before, I was too wary simply to say what I thought. Instead, I exercised the familiar technique of looking very serious, and asking the patient what *he* thought. Well, gradually it all came out, everything was part of a plot. As far as I can remember, the plot was directed towards undermining his, the patient's, character, and in a very subtle way driving him mad. There was an enormous organisation involved. For years this unfortunate young man had taken to writing down the names of those who betrayed by some (to me apparently innocent) remark that they were involved against him, that they were one of the plotters. He called it the Powey Gang, I fancy after the name of the august ringleader. By this time, the list of names, which he kept in a book, included practically all his colleagues and almost everybody with whom he had any contact during the past few years. Completely fresh contacts were not members of the gang, or not necessarily so, but it was clear to me that it would only be a question of time before they were suspect, and very soon after that they would be full-blown members. The immediate question was how to prevent my own name being added to the list prematurely. I could do this, but only for a time, by listening sympathetically to everything he said, and by being very careful not to let slip the slightest hint that I thought he might be mistaken. The thing worth studying here was the patient's emotions. The intensity of his emotional preoccupation with every detail of this delusion of his—he would actually tremble when he got warmed up to his subject, his eyes bulge and his face sweat— made it clear to me that this was his emotional life, evidently the whole of his emotional life. He had no other; every ounce of his emotional interest went into this. To try to 'cure' him of it would be attempting nothing less than to rob his id, or intinct-tension, of its only form of expression, outlet and relief. The mechanism of the mind is such that he would perforce have to resist any such attempt. You might as well put your hand over his mouth and nose and try to stop his breathing, and expect him, or the forces in him, to acquiesce in your attempt. It is just not a possibility of the laws of nature that he should acquiesce. If I had said one word against his delusions, I would immediately, automatically, have become one of the Powey Gang, and all that would have happened would have been that he lost his only friend. Hitherto, he had, so far as I knew, not taken any action against this terrible gang or this terrible world in which he lived. He was still doing his laboratory work and earning his income. I wondered how long we could maintain this practical state of affairs. I fancied it would not be for long. Nevertheless, I felt that my job was to see what could be done and for how long, until the position became too cruel, from the point of view of the patient's suffering, to maintain.

The method was twofold: firstly, to allow him to use me for the expression and discharge of this emotionally over-charged drama, and secondly, to use my position of trust and confidence to try and persuade him that the time was not yet ripe to act, not yet ripe to call the bluff of the Powey Gang. His job, I told him, was just to continue as he was, and to come whenever he liked and tell me all about it. I think we got through a year or so that way, with periodic visits to me about once a fortnight or less, and then I could see that the poor man was gradually getting worse, and that to encourage him to continue doing his ordinary laboratory work with his diseased mind was not a kindness. He was subject to chest complaints. His bronchial asthma and bronchitis were worse, he was getting thinner, and there was a risk of the supervention of organic disease. I had to betray his confidence; he was obviously too ill to co-operate, so finally I sent for his brother, who happened to be a doctor, and explained the position. He will be in a distressed state wherever he is with his delusions, but at least he will not have the added strain, and therefore suffering, of having to work and of trying to maintain his place amongst normal people.

It is such an experience as this, deeply studied, that brings to our notice the abundant minor and almost imperceptible tendencies of those around us towards comparable mental mechanisms. It is not the whole of our emotional life that can discharge itself along the primitive instinct paths. All the activities of our mental apparatus may be regarded as nothing more or less than a more recent, highly developed machinery for discharge of the surplus of our emotional energy. One might expect that the form this takes is not wholly, or all the time, accurately in strict conformity with reality and truth. Nevertheless, to the extent that it departs from such conformity do we incur adventitious sufferings for ourselves and others on every scale from family relationships to international.

I feel I must interject here a theory, or I would prefer to say a truth, of such importance for the understanding of psychology, and indeed for the understanding of the entire world of man, that the appreciation of it alone, if only I can get it across, would justify the writing and reading of this book.

The evidence for it emerges from our clinical work . . . and keeps on emerging. For instance, only recently I had a patient who was a champion tennis player. He told me that his 'addiction' to competitive tennis was practically a *compulsion*. 'Something compels me to spend my life going from tournament to tournament, from match to match. It is like a gladiatorial battle . . . to decide who shall survive and who shall be annihilated.' (Here I thought of the fighting compulsion between stags, for instance, and other male animals during the mating season.) 'It is the same with all players in all competitive games. They all feel like this: as though they are fighting for their very lives. Whatever they may pretend, I believe this is how they feel. I know I do. Otherwise I would never have become first class. Unless I play in a match, I don't want to play at all; it is not worth the trouble. I couldn't be bothered to hit the ball at all.'

This patient continued interestingly enough: 'My trouble is that I have dared to question the sense and the domination over me, and over my life, of this compulsion. If I had not questioned it, I would simply be as psychotic (mad) as the other championship players beating away at the ball.

'In practice, it's the all or nothing principle. Either you are fighting (e.g. at tennis) all the time in a life and death struggle, or else you try to pull away from the compulsion, as I have tried to do. If, through exposing it under analysis, as we have done here, as an interminable fight with father, and as a result of full insight into it, I can no longer be a victim of the illusion that my survival depends on it, and therefore am no longer the puppet of the compulsive drive, then I am "cured"!—but what have I got then? *Nothing!* I have no compulsion, no drive, no life. I might as well be dead.'

Reflections on such analytical material, of which there is an unending abundance, give one food for thinking that the whole of all of the actions of all of us in our lives are largely, if not exclusively, similarly based to this patient's compulsion to play competitive games. Whatever the source of our energies, their mode of expression is, when not along inherited instinct paths, along paths acquired and *conditioned* by the discharge pattern of our various repressed complexes. In short, it is the energy of our unconscious complexes that we are expressing all the time in forms laid down by our conditioning. Our use for so-called realities is only as toys or instruments to utilise for the playing out of the tensions of these buried pre-conditioned patterns. We *must* play them out . . . it is an essential part of the life process . . . or else the accumulating tension inside us, and its accompanying chemico-physical metabolic changes, would poison our very protoplasm, the substance of our existence. Death is when this actually happens. In other words: when our behaviour is not instinct-driven, it is being driven by what I prefer to call (in

'Irish') 'acquired instincts', or (in English) conditioned emotional patterns, identical with complicated conditioned reflexes—with their emotional accompaniments and energy-drives. It is these acquired 'instincts' together with the inherited ones that determine human behaviour no less than insect behaviour. Reality or 'truth' is utilised principally as an agent or accessory for the purposes of this life-drive. This is the theory which I cannot too strongly emphasise.

CHAPTER IX

INDIA AND MATERNITY

AFTER army training at Farnborough Camp I was sent out once again to Bombay, where I was appointed surgical specialist for the new Gerard Freeman Thomas War Hospital, and later medical officer in the fever wards. A year or so later, I was offered command of an Indian hospital train, and so my days at the war hospital came to an end. It was far more congenial to be in command of one's own unit, and very soon I became so accustomed to the routine of the work that I found there was really very little to do. I had an excellent Medical Officer in the person of a high class Brahmin who had obtained his medical qualifications at a hospital in India. He also had a junior, similarly qualified. Then there was an educated clerk and storekeeper. Apart from these three, the rest of the staff were unable to speak English. There was an enormous bearded, soldierly man called the havildar, the equivalent of a British sergeant-major, and under him some six or eight elegant Sikh soldiers. They were the ward orderlies, trained for the job, most dignified gentlemen, all with beards and beautiful long hair which they spent a good part of their mornings in dressing. Then there were the four mathas or sweepers (the untouchables) four or five cooks, and in addition to these, my own personal cook and servant attendant, and a whole batch of railway workers under the charge of a European foreman. These last occupied a compartment comparable to the brake van at the end of the train, and I saw little or nothing of them.

We would load up with Indian troops from a hospital in Bombay, and take them to various parts of the country, sometimes as far as Lahore, Lucknow, Secunderabad, Madras, Bangalore, or further south to the foothill station for Ootacumund, and eastwards even to Calcutta. The journey commonly occupied two or three days and nights across India, sometimes we would rest for twenty-four hours at our destination, and practically always return empty. It was during these long empty journeys, finding nothing to do and getting tired of reading, that I took to amusing myself by composing verse. Finally I made it into a fairly practised hobby, but I doubt whether my inspiration was sufficiently poetical for anything of permanent value to emerge.

During a hot evening, with the train rolling interminably through the Rajputana desert, gazing out of my carriage window at the wonderful tropical sunset, I wrote:

> The land deserted, dreary:
> Afar the setting sun
> Sinks, red-eyed and weary:
> The Eastern day is done.

Then, after a few indifferent verses, being somewhat overcome by my own sentiments:

> O love, do not bereave me
> When all things so distress . . .

I did not like the emotion I was moved to express, and stopped. I had lately received distressing news of Winifred's worsening condition. My feelings were too vivid and current to bear expression.

In the later evening under the electric lights in my saloon, sitting alone at dinner, waited on hand and foot by my Indian staff, I would again be lost in thought. Occasionally hosts of insects of infinite variety found their way through the ventilator to interest and annoy, often committing suicide in the soup. There are more species of insects (half a million have been described) than of all other living creatures put together, and one has to be in the tropics to appreciate the fact. Thoughtfully observing a little fellow with particularly bright pea-green wings, and made morbidly introspective by my solitude, I wrote:

> O little green fly, sitting on my plate,
> So blissfully to every danger blind,
> O fairy sprite, unthoughtful of your fate,
> Let me just creep into your tiny mind.

Your universe all circumscribed and bound
Within a circle of instinctive deed!
You boldly flit where food is to be found
And, seated on the brink of death, you feed.

. . . . .

And, little green fly, what in truth are we,
Who deem you wingéd Folly, foolish sprite.
Blindly as you we fall to Destiny:
Blindly as you we vanish into Night.

So life on the Ambulance Train had its contemplative and sentimental moments. . . .

A medical incident in the course of this work with Indians
may be worth recording. My chief Assistant Medical Officer, the
Brahmin, was responsible for medical attention to all members of
the train staff, and rather jealous of his command in this respect.
I was supposed to be too high and mighty to have anything to do
with such little matters as staff sick parade or the illnesses of
the Indians under me. One day he reported that one of the sweepers
was not very well, and he had taken him off duty. I asked what was
the matter with him, and he replied that he was, 'Just a little bit
out of sorts.' 'Well,' I said, 'you are quite confident about your
ability to look after him?' He was. I thought nothing more about
this matter until six weeks later when, in the course of signing
his letters in reply to correspondence and dealing with office
matters in general, there appeared amongst the pile of papers a
blue form for the purpose of admitting a patient to the large
Indian military hospital in Bombay. I looked at it and noticed
the name of the sweeper. I asked the Brahmin assistant, 'Has this
man been ill in bed on the train all these weeks?' 'Yes, sir.' 'What
is the matter with him? What's the diagnosis?' He pointed to the
form; there was the diagnosis plainly written, 'Debility'. I said:
'Well, you had better bring him along here and let me have a
look at him.' I could not understand the enormous length of time
that elapsed between this order and the appearance of the man,
until I heard, and caught sight of, him being carried by four
attendants (apparently he could not walk) through the narrow

corridor of the train to be placed on a berth in a small ward. When they had finally got him ready, I came into the ward with the Indian assistant and looked at the man. He was almost a skeleton, just skin and bone. I said to my assistant, hitherto regarded by me as extraordinarily capable and trustworthy: 'What is his temperature?' He had never taken it. We secured a thermometer, and he was astonished to find that the temperature was nearly 101°. I then said: 'What is this rash on his body?' His eyes popped, and he stared closely. He had never noticed any rash, but he could see it now, practically all over the man's body. Then feeling his shin bones, I said: 'What are these lumps on his bones?' These, too, had not been observed. I pointed out lumps and swellings in his groins, under his armpits, and conspicuously in his neck. They were glands, swollen and tender. I told the man to put out his tongue, and it looked like a map of Europe! His Medical Officer had never noticed that. Next I got him to open his mouth, and we looked inside with a torch. It was full of irregular ulcers, especially on his fauces. I said to the Medical Officer: 'What is the diagnosis?' He still did not know. 'Well,' I said, 'roll back his foreskin.' And there was the primary chancre as large as life!

My next move was the one upon which I pride myself. I asked: 'Who is this man's greatest friend on the train?' I received the answer: 'Your own cook, sir.' I said: 'Bring him along.' They did, and on exposing his glans penis, there was an almost identical sore! Thus we had two blue forms, and I crossed out the word 'debility' and wrote in the diagnosis for them both, 'syphilis'. It is the only time in my life that I have seen a person practically in process of dying from this curable disease. Both men were completely cured and resumed their duties, though this was decades before the days of penicillin.

In due course I was, despite my unworthiness, appointed C.O. of the prize hospital train of India called the British 'A' Ambulance Train. About that time the Great War ended; but before we had been very long in Bombay, awaiting embarkation to England, the Afghan War broke out. Our demobilisation plans were instantly stopped, and my train, complete with staff, was one of the first units to be sent up to Rawalpindi for service between there and Peshawar. It was early summer, and climatically the hottest experience of my life. The temperature on the train used regularly to reach 120° in the shade. Between Rawalpindi and Peshawar we travelled only at night; it was considered too hot for survival to be on the train in the day time, with the summer sun blazing down upon it.

One morning in Rawalpindi I happened to tell my young friend, the Railway Transport Officer, an incident I had had with a European engine driver. He said :'Oh yes, I know all about it; he has already filed a complaint against you. Would you like to see it?' I was a little taken aback, and accompanied him into his office on the station. There he took out a great file about the size of a large book, and read me out the long letter of complaint from the engine driver, already received and filed. With a sudden feeling of awful misgiving, I said to him: 'And what is all this other great mass of papers?' 'Oh,' he said, 'in this file they are all complaints against you.' I ran through them and saw reports of incidents which I had practically forgotten. Literally there were dozens of these letters. I remarked, a little bewildered: 'I had no idea of this, I have not heard of one of these things.' The R.T.O. replied: 'No, and you won't. Colonel So-and-So likes you and the official letters you send up almost every day, reporting things that are wrong with the railway and so on. He stamps them all and sends them up to Simla. If you were a regular and stayed long enough, you'd get promoted to high office. When he gets these complaints, he just roars with laughter and says, "Who'd have thought it of Berg? He is such a quiet, well-behaved chap." ' I am ashamed to say that I wrote most of my letters as a pastime for literary practice.

It was partly by dint of my aggressive letters, and partly by taking advantage of my position as a temporary Medical Officer who could demand immediate demobilisation whenever he liked, as the war for which I had enlisted was over, that by this time I had managed to get my salary pushed up to equal that of a permanent colonel in the R.A.M.C. In consequence, as I was saving quite a bit of money, I was in no particular hurry to return to England. Thus, I did not resist my being appointed Medical Officer to a large hospital in Deolali. I secured a house for my mother amongst the officers' married quarters, and worked for several months there until I found that the regular Army Colonel in charge was becoming increasingly jealous of my privileged position and endeavouring to give me all the hard work in the place. Soon after this, I got leave and interviewed the authorities in Bombay, and arranged for my return to England and demobilisation. This was nearly a year after the European war was over.

In the meantime, my sister had got married to an Army chaplain in Madras. My brother had long since returned to his wife and family in London (he married when a student). My family and I had, a couple of years earlier, experienced almost the worst tragedy imaginable. My father had died suddenly, all in a day, from acute ptomaine poisoning, while I was alone with him in the house in Bombay, at a time when my sister was near death's door in a hospital in Lahore. My mother had left us with the servants to be near my sister. I do not wish to go into the details of that painful and harrowing time. I could not bring myself to wire or write the news of the tragedy to my already anxious mother. Instead, I got leave and went personally to Lahore. There, I found that under the leading I.M.S. doctors of the place, a major and a colonel, my sister had encountered a succession of various diagnoses. The first had been appendicitis, the second malaria, and there had been several others. She was now in her third week of illness, desperately ill and weak, and still running a fluctuating temperature. She had very narrowly escaped being subjected to a major operation. I sat by her bedside, studied her temperature chart, and looked at her. I had to avoid giving any impression to the nurses that I was at all professionally interested in her. Nevertheless, that evening I was called in to the Sister's room and informed by her that Major So-and-So, in charge of my sister, had left an official message for me. It was to the effect that my sister did not appear to be making much progress in that hospital, and now that I was present to supervise, would I please remove her to a hill station immediately. In fact, he had given orders for an ambulance to be there next morning for that purpose. I said to the Sister: 'You can cancel the ambulance. I will write a letter to Major So-and-So.' At least I had the sense not to give a verbal message but with the emotional violence of youth and the fact that I had had as much stress as I could endure, I began my letter by saying: 'I have had your message. I will not remove my sister from this hospital as she is suffering from paratyphoid fever and would die on the journey.' Of course, it was a bomb. Major So-and-So would have murdered me if he could have got away with it. I may say that nowadays in my maturity I would behave differently. I would not be so introverted and hide behind pen and paper. I would go and see the man personally wherever he lived and have it out with him, or rather deal with him according to his psychological requirements. When eventually my sister was convalescing some weeks later, and I did take her to Simla, I was informed immediately by the doctor she was placed under that her urine was still full of bacillus paratyphoid B. Perhaps it was not for nothing that I had worked for so many months in charge of typhoid wards. One could almost smell out typhoid and paratyphoid fever. Somebody there had been foolish enough to entrain several of his cases, and some of those in the third week had actually died on their way to the ambulance train.

My mother was left with my sister in India, preparatory to following me, while I embarked on the s.s. *Patricia*. When I arrived in London, I proceeded to obtain lodgings for myself and to rejoin St. Thomas's Hospital to put in the necessary year of further study in order to sit for my university degree (M.B., B.S.) which I had deferred on account of the war emergency. I soon stepped into the temporary job of House Physician, but having grown accustomed to being in charge of large numbers of sick myself, and my opinion and prescriptions passing unquestioned, I did not take kindly to the junior role of having to give professional precedence to medical registrars or resident assistant physicians, who were at liberty to prescribe and to give orders above my head. There seemed to be very little work to do, and absolutely no responsibility. I felt it was largely a waste of time, and that I could do much better with complete liberty to interest myself and to study as I wished. I was actually in the bath of our out-patient cloakroom in Casualty when in walked a young officer in uniform, a Thomas's man, whom I had met in India. He had arrived by the boat after mine. The first thing he said to me was: 'Do you know how I can get a job in this hospital?' On the spur of the moment I said: 'Yes.' He said: 'What job?' I said: 'Mine.' He said: 'When?' I said: 'Now,' and with that we promptly arranged the transfer . . . and I was free again.

There were a few things that impressed me very much on my return to London. One was an early experience of walking over

Westminster Bridge in a moderately thick fog on a rather wet, uncomfortable day. I found myself wondering why on earth anybody lived here. I had just come from sunny climes and wide open spaces. Another impression, perhaps at the same time, was when wandering through the West End I felt I must somehow have lost my bearings and got into the slums, it all seemed so cramped, dismal and dirty. Afterwards I confirmed that it must have been —not Soho—but actually 'magnificent' Piccadilly Circus that I was in at that moment during that dingy day, for I distinctly remember noticing the statue of Eros. However, the spring soon came and I was usually in very high spirits just at that period of my life. I was most excited at finding myself so close to so many people. In India, everything had seemed so wide, far apart, and distant. But here in London one got into buses and sat close to perfect strangers, people one had never seen before and would not see again, and all these faces crowded around one were to me of enormous, stimulating interest. I even found a great delight in going to Selfridge's; and the thrill of going up and down in crowded lifts! If one is young and goes about smiling at everybody, it is surprising how many smiles one gets in return. Perhaps it was a bit of my father's debonair attitude which had been so embarrassing to me at a younger age. The mood of happiness and freedom seemed to be shared by most people around me, possibly it was a general reaction after the war; a reaction which I have not noticed at all, apart from Victory Day activities, after the second world war. However, I remember what a delight it was to 'get off' with all and sundry wherever I went.

One of the branches of my professional work which I had not kept up-to-date during my five years of national service had been midwifery and gynaecology. I realised that this would be particularly important if I 'had a go' at general practice, which I wanted to take up both because of my interest in that branch of medical work and because of my complete ignorance of it. I felt one would never be a 'proper doctor' until one had gone out into the world and met the public in the role of their individual practitioner, not a mere medical cipher, but with a full assignment of responsibility and humanity. It was partly to prepare for this that I had returned to resume my studies and to make them up-to-date. First on the list was to get abreast again of this special department.

Therefore it was not long before I obtained the post of Resident Medical Officer at what was then called the York Road Lying-In Hospital. It was only a stone's throw from St. Thomas's, and I believe I must have heard of the vacancy and got the appointment through St. Thomas's.

My position there suited me down to the ground. There were several dozen beds, and a very large ante-natal out-patient department; and the glory of it was that I was the one and only Resident Medical Officer. The visiting gynaecologists did not trouble me much as they seemed so rarely on the premises. Some of the senior sisters at the hospital were very knowledgeable people, rather conscious and a bit jealous of their superior knowledge in the face of the young Resident Medical Assistant placed, in a sense, officially above them. As in all human relationships, it would seem that tact was the most necessary requirement. I was quite ready to recognise that these sisters had been doing this work, some of them for nearly a quarter of a century, whereas I, whatever I read up in books, was practically a newcomer. Nevertheless, I always felt, however much of a newcomer I was, that I possessed more general sagacity, and would not be likely to let other people have their way unless they could convince me, and I was quite ready to be convinced, that their way was better than my personal opinion.

From the large ante-natal clinic, selected expectant mothers were admitted, sometimes weeks before labour was due, on account of various medical or surgical abnormalities. A fair proportion were admitted on account of the formation of their pelvis being prejudicial to, or impossible for, normal birth at full term. Nowadays, I expect a larger number of these would be treated to caesarian section, but it may be at that time caesarian was not the one hundred per cent safe operation that it is to-day, and a good many inductions were the rule, in spite of the fact that a fair number of these seemed, quite unaccountably, to result in a still-birth. In actual fact, the result of the application of these principles was that almost every afternoon I personally had to perform about two or three inductions. It was quite a new experience for me, having just come from five years' surgical and medical attendance, exclusively upon adult males, suddenly to find myself engaged in this particular form of work. One of the sisters would give the anaesthetic, officially under my responsibility, the patient would be put in the lithotomy position, that is to say with knees raised and legs apart, held either by the crutches of the operating table, or by nurses while she lay at the end of a bed. Another nurse would hold a bright, shielded spot lamp over my head, while I, with Castor peering over one of my shoulders and Pollux over the other (my two very pretty female medical students whom I had christened at sight 'The Heavenly Twins') would perform the operation of induction, demonstrating every stage and movement and explaining it to them in full detail as I did so.

The fact that I was often called out at night on this job did not worry me. There was always something of interest, if not actually exciting, and I felt I was a part of the hospital and a part of the work. I very soon came to understand all these mothers, expectant and otherwise. I grew to understand how they looked at their condition and situation, and the way they felt. There is little doubt that the state of pregnancy commonly makes a woman more vegetative, more contented and comfortable, like a broody hen. I think it is as though her body had at last achieved its aim. Whatever sort of wily, 'bitchy', paranoid or other variety of vixen she may have been before pregnancy, in her pregnant state all this seems to go, and she is just a contented, comfortable, feminine, motherly creature. Perhaps I saw them all at their best. Anyway, in the presence of these real, fundamental facts of life— happy facts because most mothers, whatever they allege, are deeply satisfied with their condition—any adolescent, fetishistic or sexual interests become not only unworthy but completely nonsensical. I have thought at times that perhaps it is a pity that fetishists and various perverts could not be treated to a form of therapy which included their familiarisation with these facts of life, by, for instance, living in this sort of hospital and having to do what I had to do; but of course my deeper knowledge of patients and their psychopathology tells me that conscious-level observations of this sort cannot cure the real pervert. At the most, they may act as a corrective to such tendencies in the normal person only.

During my work at that hospital I developed a great sympathy for all these mothers; maybe that was not difficult, as most of them were young, but I think my sympathy extended to all women, not excepting the elderly sisters who were not even mothers, though always it was chiefly with the patients—before, during and after their childbirth. The atmosphere in this hospital was naturally much happier than that in any other sort of hospital, whether one is in the medical wards or surgical. After all, an ordinary hospital is for sick people, for morbid states, whereas this, on the contrary, was for the triumph of a natural process, even if some of the patients were not undergoing it quite naturally. I am glad to reflect that I did not develop the god complex, only too frequently seen amongst accoucheurs and gynaecologists and evidently fostered by their dealing exclusively with women who, out of their anxiety and out of the intimate exposure of themselves, cling to them as though they were omnipotent saviours. I may have gone so far as to begin to feel as though these people, the mothers even more than the infants, were all my babies. I am sure there was a sort of transference here, for I always put their welfare before my own, day or night, without regard for any sacrifice of my leisure or rest and could not have taken more pains on their behalf. Probably it was more satisfying for me to attend to them than to do anything else whatsoever. It was indeed the best training for general medical practice, because, I was subsequently to learn, that it is just such an emotional attitude which makes one the ideal medical practitioner.

It is probably inadvisable to become a doctor unless one can feel something like this towards one's patients, and if one does feel like this, it is patently impossible to have any other important interest in life. One is sunk in the thing, like Newton in his mathematics, and Darwin in his biology. The essence of this quality of interest is that it takes precedence over self. One forgets to have one's meals or one's sleep if there is an emergency, perhaps in the same way that one would forget these things if a child or loved member of one's family were in distress and in urgent need of one's help. Perhaps it could be said that one acquires such a large family that there will never be any time to attend to anything else. I dare say the appeal of this sort of thing is an extremely healthy and natural one. A mother who resigns herself to nature's laws is in a comparable position, forever giving birth, suckling and tending an ever-growing family. I would not say that she must necessarily be harassed; she will just be absorbed

H

CHAPTER X

GENERAL PRACTICE

M Y job in the York Road Lying-In Hospital came to an end. I had still to do the necessary medical and surgical work for my university degree. In the meantime, my mother had arrived from India, and the best we could do to start with was to secure a room for her in the same apartment house as myself. Our money was very limited, she having little more than twelve hundred pounds scraped up from the wreck of my father's investments, the wreck which terminated our stay in Switzerland, and I having only a few hundred pounds saved from the latter part of my military service, and a government educational grant, on account of interrupted academic studies, amounting to one hundred and fifty pounds a year to last for one year only. Nevertheless, it did not occur to me for a moment to have the slightest financial anxiety.

I negotiated the M.B., B.S., but I must admit that I found this examination more of a strain than I had ever found any other. I grew so tired during the seemingly endless practical work and viva voces, probably through having already exhausted myself with the interminable written papers; or it may have been that life had temporarily unsettled me for such concentrated study and such a high standard of examination work. One afternoon, towards the end of a gruelling three weeks, I was doing the practical bacteriology examination. The specimens to be diagnosed included a milky fluid which one had to examine first as a hanging drop specimen under the microscope before drying it and staining it for oil immersion. I had completed this and the other nine or ten tasks an hour before the end of the three hours allowed, and written up my results in the little paper book provided. There was nothing else to do; I knew one could not leave until after the viva, so I perched myself up on the pathology counter beside the sink and microscope, so that I could view the large hall from the fairly generous cubicle designed for each candidate, smoked a cigarette, and swung my legs. Presently, a little man in a dirty khaki overall with slightly dishevelled hair darted up behind me from the depths of the hall, and asked me if I had finished. Taking him for a lab.

boy, I hardly bothered to answer; I was tired. Then he started asking me what I considered to be a lot of unnecessary questions: 'Did you diagnose your hanging drop specimen?' I nodded carelessly. He said: 'What was it?' I said: 'Diphtheroid.' He said: 'Diphtheroid? Why, what makes you think it is not diphtheria?' I said: 'It's alive. I don't suppose the examiners would be such bloody fools as to throw a lot of live diphtheria bacilli about amongst all these students.' He then asked what I thought was his first intelligent question: 'How would you distinguish?' I said carelessly: 'Guinea pig.' With that he went off, and I continued to wait. Finally, an official came along and collected my papers. I said: 'But I have not had my viva yet.' He said: 'Oh yes you have, an hour ago.' And then I realised! Anyway, I got through. Perhaps at the final M.B. the examiners do not concern themselves with peculiarities of character.

As after every important examination for which I had sat, my mother, unless she were away in India, was waiting for me at the foot of the auspicious steps that led from the Imperial Institute building in South Kensington. Her face was always solicitous, anxious and enquiring. I believe she suffered more tension and anxiety on my behalf than I felt myself. I am sure it is this devotion and empathy on the part of a mother, at any rate in the absence of any comparable interest from another person, that make a boy, girl, man and woman whatever they become in life. Though I was now not more than a few years from thirty, I felt, particularly since my father's death, that my mother and I were one. It was not altogether comfortable having a person a generation older than oneself, and one's mother at that, as one's closest and perhaps only really intimate associate. But fate had evidently so decreed it, and it was quite obvious that there was no other comparable alliance for my mother, so I must console myself with the enormous advantages it brought, though I was not yet sure of the best way to handle the undoubted disadvantages. There were, of course, by that time a fair number of young women ready to enlighten me. As is not unusual, that side of my life, which certainly did exist, was a thing completely concealed from, and I hoped unsuspected by, this dear, devoted lady, whose whole being was one great love of me.

In those five years of enforced extroversion and generally

confused rubbing-of-shoulders with all and sundry, my ideas had
undergone some modification. I was now coming round to the view
that before specialising in what to me, at that time, must have
seemed like a sort of philosophical study of the mind and of mental
phenomena, I must first experience the life of the general practitioner. Surely such an experience was far too rich emotionally and
intellectually to be side-stepped altogether. I guessed one would
never do it once one started specialisation. The first important
item on such a programme is, or should be, to do a series of locums
for general practitioners. It was usual to secure these through
the agency of the Head Porter, to whom it seemed that all St.
Thomas's men in general practice were in the habit of applying.

The first place I went to was a large practice in Peterborough,
where I met an extremely efficient and fairly busy man and his
wife. I can still remember the extraordinary degree of enthusiasm,
keenness and hard work with which I tackled this, my first 'real'
job. In my eagerness, it seems I gave everybody far more than
their money's worth, far more than they had ever expected from
a general practitioner. The result was that when the doctor
returned after three weeks, he found that instead of his practice
losing clientele, which is commonly expected from abandoning
it to a locum, it had actually increased. This man was reputed
never to have taken a holiday before since he started the practice
ten years previously, but in less than six months after this experience, he was pressing for me to do another three weeks' locum
for him. I worked for him three times within that first year.
I also, between these times, did a locum for his partner who had
a fairly large country practice in an attractive village of two or
three thousand inhabitants and in half a dozen out-lying villages.
This man, who was older, subsequently tried to sell me his practice,
to which he was extraordinarily devoted, making the terms such
that I would not have to put down any capital, but would be able
to buy the goodwill and the freehold of his house, property and
orchard out of a small proportion of the income of the practice.
He kept the offer open for years. At one stage of my life, this
tempted me, but only slightly. It was too far from London. I felt
it would have been quite a delightful life, but of too vegetative
a nature for the energies I then possessed.

Apart from these isolated locum jobs, I arranged with the St.

Thomas's porter-agency to do a continuous series of locums all over the country, going straight from one to another, covering a period of nearly six months. I rightly thought that such a training would break me in to general practice in an adequate way, and tell me the sort of practice that would suit me best, if I did decide to go in for it for a longer period of time. The series began in the early summer with my going to a practice in Kenilworth, Warwickshire. This was what I subsequently described as a 'silly ass practice'. The practitioner insisted upon giving me a couple of days' 'tuition' before he departed. He and all his clients appeared to be very rich. He had a great Daimler car, driven by a liveried chauffeur, and we used to roll out to great houses, often inhabited by titled people, in big estates.

Well, we visited many important people, some of them admittedly with quite serious illnesses. There was, for instance, a gentleman in a wonderful bedroom with a lovely balcony overlooking his estate. He had advanced tuberculosis, presumably too advanced for sanatorium cure abroad. One's function was to sit leisurely in a large chair near the foot of the bed, and discuss the latest racing news. I had the privilege of listening in to some of this discussion, and wondering whether I would ever make a practitioner. Perhaps I did not yet quite realise that a person with serious and fatal illness, like every other case of organic disease, is in real need of psychotherapy, and that my own method of administering it might not include the racing news, but might be just as meritorious for all that. Eventually, the doctor departed with his family on holiday, and left me in the care of chauffeur and staff of servants.

It was while I was a locum at a practice in Brixton that the sort of medical incident occurred with which locums and assistants are only too familiar. The practitioner had on his panel-list most of the girls working at the large local drapery and other stores (since largely destroyed by bombing in the last war) in the High Street. Amongst the clientele at the evening surgery, one of these girls, perhaps a little older than the majority, had been a fairly regular attendant. She had complained, and kept on complaining, of abdominal discomforts, and I felt she had done her best to simulate appendicitis. I had therefore made it my business to make quite sure of what was the matter with her, and had come to the

definite conclusion that there was absolutely nothing organic the
matter, and that the most she could possibly be suffering from was
constipation, probably psychogenic. Also I had suspected that she
was solicitous for the special attention of the young-man locum. It
was fortunate that I was in this confident position, for one night
after evening surgery, the managing director of the company
employing her elected to telephone me. He was very brusque and
dictatorial; presumably he knew that I was only a young locum, and
felt that intimidation would be easy. I did not bother to ask myself or him what his special interest might be in the young lady.
His attitude was that he did not believe I was competent to handle
the case. Surely I should have admitted her to hospital for operation, etc. What did I propose to do about it? I said on the phone:
'I will tell you what I will do. I will be round there in ten minutes.
Will you ask the nurse in charge of the dormitories (where the
girls slept) to have a jug of hot water, a jug of cold water, and a
basin ready.' In ten minutes I was there with my bag, some soft
soap, and a Higginson's syringe. There was a great hoo-ha. All
the girls had been swept away out of sight, except this one, clad
in a nightdress. On my instructions, the nurse laid her on her
side. It did not take me many minutes to pump in a pint and a half
of warm, soapy water enema. I departed immediately and left them
to it. Never did I hear one word of complaint from the managing
director or any other official again. There is often a great advantage
in knowing, and in being perfectly confident in one's knowledge.
The girl was absolutely and completely and, as far as I was concerned, permanently cured.

Of course, one realises that such an attitude is purely superficial,
however appropriate or necessary it may be to the convenience of
a busy practitioner. One realises that people who are inclined
to pester are doing so for perfectly adequate causes (there is
no effect without a cause directly and proportionately related to
it), though the cause may not be the organic disease or the complaint which they allege. It may, nevertheless, in a sense be just
as important, or more important. I expect this young woman,
and the legions of which she is only one, have a need which their
life is not satisfying or even promising any prospect of satisfying.
Perhaps she had outgrown the initial excitement and unconscious anticipations which were keeping her younger associates

healthy, happy and giggly, and was reaching a stage in life when it was becoming obvious to her that shop-assistantship was not the answer she wanted, and also obvious to her that she could no longer anticipate or see a way out. On account of the habit of repression, it is conceivable that she was not sufficiently or clearly conscious of her real needs. She dumbly and blindly came to a young man and complained. Perhaps after all I did not treat her as kindly as I might have done to-day. The self-confidence of the young, even when seemingly justified, is not always so clever, comprehending or sympathetic as that of the more mature and experienced. On reflection it occurs to me that this and similar behaviour must have been an over-compensation for shyness, modesty, and a more natural introversion.

Perhaps it would not be out of place to mention here a non-medical incident that occured while I was at this same locum, if only to show that medical practice was not the whole of one's life (though it very nearly was).

Sylvia came to see me. Sylvia was a sweetly pretty young lady of some private means with whom I had considered myself in love for several years. (My mother said I strove to warm only the cold-hearted). For a long while our contact had been largely by correspondence, as she travelled much, on my part voluminous letters pouring out almost everything, with a predilection for hilarity— I felt hilariously happy while writing to her; hers a short formal paragraph or two in reply. A gradual cooling process had been in operation for some time, but on this occasion Sylvia had taken the initiative and come to see me. I found her in the lounge of this old-fashioned house, looking wistfully out of the window. She was sad; and actually a tear trickled down her cheek. Sylvia, of all people! One would not have dreamt it possible.

With some difficulty I wrung the story out of her. For three years she had been in love with a young man in South Africa, apparently imagining that one day they would wed, and now she had received a letter from him announcing his engagement to a girl in Capetown. She wept. It did not take long to proffer the appropriate advice. I said to her: 'From what I know of you, which apparently is even less than I realised, it is a safe bet that this man has no conception that you were ever in love with him at all, so your clear duty is to write and tell him so immediately, and take the consequences.'

This she did. The consequences were that he broke his engagement in Africa and came post-haste to meet her in London. Perhaps
a disengaged man was less attractive to Sylvia than an engaged
man for, when she met him, one look was enough. Sylvia was free
again.

I was rather dull-witted in appreciating this young lady's
psychology. She was always in love with the boy-friend who was
furthest away—three thousand miles at least. My turn came finally
some years later, when she was travelling in India. Then I began
to receive the real Sylvia—volumes of rather shy but heart-felt
out-pourings. But it was all too late. Absence never made my
heart grow fonder. I realised that I had attached a phantasy to this
beautiful feminine picture simply because it was feminine and
beautiful. Her quiet reserve had facilitated the process. But the
revelations of these long letters brought a reality-corrective to
bear upon the relationship.

Where love was concerned, Sylvia would always be distant in
space and time. In fact, she waited till all her passionate potentialities had cooled with age, and eventually married an elderly
nobleman who died soon after. She had secured immunity from
sexuality and had instead an empty title and full purse. To her
credit I am sure she had planned neither. She is still roaming the
world. Maybe roamers are those who have grown tired of 'waiting
for Godot' and have decided to take action and search for him.

About this time with my mother's connivance and help I began
to look round for a practice for myself. The first practice I found
(at Enfield) was not bad, but also it was not good. What tired
me most was sitting in the surgery during surgery hours waiting
for the next patient to come in. That was an experience which I had
never had in any of the locums I had done, and I found it a little
depressing. There were, at the most, five or six visits a day, and I
found it is just as easy to spend the whole day doing a handful of
visits as to get through twenty or thirty in the same time. It is only
pressure of work behind the general practitioner that makes him
go quickly, at least that was so in my case. Possibly I took more
pleasure in actually being with patients than most practically-
minded doctors would have done, and in consequence gave them
more time than was economically sound. Certainly economics,
during this experience, were far from good.

Eventually, on this account, I found myself a practice (in North London) which was a very different proposition ; but like a lot of idealists or semi-idealists, I seem to have been reluctant to accept the fact that the fundamental basis of our reality life is economics. (I am not referring to the conventional pretence that it is not, for I was never hypocritical). Such a recognition was to some extent being forced upon me. After having lived almost imperceptibly a little beyond our income at Enfield, my mother and I could now raise only seven hundred and fifty pounds towards the necessary capitation fee, but I appealed to the British Legion, which professed to have the rehabilitation of ex-officers at heart, and to my amazement, they readily lent me two hundred and fifty pounds practically on trust. At the end of one year I had paid it back completely. I do not think I ever again saved as much as two hundred and fifty pounds in a year, although the practice steadily increased. There is no doubt that I was carried along more by my emotional interest in the work and the patients than by any economic considerations. I could not get the idea into my head, as apparently my predecessor and many doctors in the neighbourhood certainly did, that one's main object in busying oneself all day was to collect half-crowns as quickly as possible. I have even heard of one local doctor who was said to look for the fee on the mantelpiece before he looked towards the patient, and Dr. Fisher himself, this delightful, jolly, red-faced little man who had sold me the practice and who did such an incredible amount of work, also, on close observation, gave the impression that his extraordinary busyness was greatly stimulated by the ever-increasing amount of money he was collecting. Maybe this is inevitable with those whose 'reality sense' is greater than their emotional satisfaction in the work. Perhaps we should not be too hard on them, for after all, every business man is largely, if not primarily, concerned in increasing the profits and dividends of his business, and this does not necessarily mean that he is producing shoddy goods. In my case, the emotional absorption with the work and the patients made it positively difficult for me to make the earning of the money anything but of secondary importance.

However, I think my theory was vaguely (and I still think there is something, if not everything, in it) that if one is interested and busily engaged and the economic principle is not wholly absent, one will probably do better than the skin-flinting type of business man. If one is going to be primarily a business man, why do the medical work at all, why not be a sort of company promoter, buying practices and putting real doctors in to work them for the company. That is the sort of thing that our Ministry of Health is now doing. When the business affairs of my practice did not seem to be going as well as I would have expected from the amount of work I was doing, when there was any economic situation that demanded my attention and worried me, I often thought: 'I wish to goodness this practice were being run by a business man and I had nothing to do with the economic side of it, but was just being paid a salary and knew that it would meet all my needs and ensure solvency.' I felt it was too much to expect anybody to be an artist, as it were, a scientist or a devotee to his patients, and at the same time to be everlastingly worrying and juggling with pounds, shillings and pence.

It was some little time before it dawned on me that the half of all the private fees which I was paying to Dr. Fisher really amounted to the total profit on all the private patients. At that time, people paid half a crown in the surgery. Everybody expected to come out with at least one bottle of medicine, properly dispensed, corked, labelled, and wrapped in paper and sealing-waxed. I had to pay a dispenser to do all these things, and in addition had to pay for the contents of the bottle of medicine, the cost of the bottle, the cork, the label, the wrapping and the sealing wax. I had to pay all this out of my half of the fee the patient paid, that is to say, out of one and threepence; but the tragedy of it all was that I discovered that, under the agreement, I was paying, in addition, income tax on the whole of the half-crown. I think I must have been there a year and a half at least before I figured out that this agreement, so far as the private-patient-side of the practice was concerned, was a dead loss.

It was not many months after I had installed myself in the house, and settled down with my mother, that I began to feel that this part of London was a bit dull and dingy. There were too many people living too close together. I liked them all well enough, but was I industriously burying myself in a slum? I fancy that what sustained me was that I was acquiring, as it were, a new love, a new lover. Perhaps these intimate soul-mate endeavours were doomed to difficulties and disappointments, but my new love on the contrary, perhaps because I was less possessive, less full of expectations and demands, grew and multiplied apace. It was a composite person, its numbers were legion, it consisted of the thousands of patients of my practice, ever-increasing numerically and in depth of professional and mental intimacy. Did I really need anything more, anything more personal? Perhaps not very badly at that time; after all, I had my mother also. Although I did not talk much to her, and certainly kept most of my thoughts and interests to myself, she somehow stood as a living symbol of all that had been 'me' up to the present time; and of all that in the present time I had passed on to this emotional, professional marriage, to these hundreds and thousands of families.

The position in a medical practice is that one is consulted or called in when people are in trouble, in distress, or in some disturbed and unhappy condition. The contact, if one appreciates it, is immediately of an emotional nature in which the practitioner's role is something like that of the good fairy, if not the ambassador of God Himself. Many is the time that I have rung the bell at a house I had not previously visited, and some middle-aged woman has opened the door and scowled at me, full of latent, ill-concealed hostility, evidently thinking that I was the rent-collector or some traveller. I have simply said the magic word 'Doctor' and watched with interest her hostility melt visibly, her face become wreathed in welcoming smiles, as she eagerly gave me the freedom of the house, and gratefully accepted and valued my ministrations to her child or husband. The circumstances of the situation no doubt provide the easiest and best form of emotional contact with the best side of everybody's character, devoid of all defences in one's presence. From the word 'go' one gets in, as it were, on the ground floor.

There was a great deal of work to be done, and I recognised from the start that the essence of the situation was to be kind, friendly and benevolent to everybody, never to show impatience or to lose one's temper, to be swift if necessary and to get on with things, but never to appear unduly worried, at least not to one's patients. Whatever affects of one's own one had to discharge, it was most inappropriate to discharge them at the expense of people who had called one in to relieve their anxiety and their tension; to use one for the discharge of *their* affects.

From this distant perspective, it is not altogether easy to remember commonplace medical incidents. There were dozens every
day. On rare occasions, I have actually seen as many as a hundred
patients a day, but fortunately this was not the rule. One was busy
enough, nevertheless. In spite of my busyness, I am sure that the
people in that neighbourhood had never before, and possibly never
since, experienced such painstaknig care and attention in return for
their paltry payment, or without the paltry payment, for I treated
panel patients and even paupers with equally unremitting care.
Perhaps it was partly ignorance or lack of gumption on my part,
and of course the hospital training had something to do with it;
one had been taught always to examine every patient very
thoroughly, no matter what his complaint. It took me a long time
to learn which patients not to examine. My examinations were unnecessarily thorough. One thing I could never endure was to allow
a new visit to remain untended. I had to be there as soon as possible,
perhaps to relieve my own anxiety or curiosity, and this irrespective of whether the patient were paying, panel or pauper.

One summer, a middle-aged man in my surgery produced some
newspaper cuttings and showed them to me. I could not understand
why he was wasting my time, asking me to read them. Evidently
there had been some correspondence in the newspapers; some
people had written letters complaining of discrimination on the
part of their doctors because they were panel patients. It seemed
that doctors were reluctant to visit them at all, or else put them last
on their visiting lists, and often they were not seen till the next day
or later. This man then showed me the cutting of a letter which had
been published in reply to this. It was documentary; in complete
contradiction to all these assertions, the writer stated that *his*
panel doctor had visited him on Christmas Day, on a bicycle, in the
midst of the heaviest snow storm that he had ever seen. He and his
wife had been looking out of the bedroom window, and down the
thickly snow-covered and deserted street they had seen a man
plodding along on a bicycle with a little bag swinging from the
lamp bracket in front. They had said to each other: 'Who is that
poor fellow out in this snow storm?' Imagine their amazement when
the 'poor fellow' stopped at their house and rang their bell. Said the
patient to me: 'As I told the newspaper in my letter, it was my
panel doctor, and all I had wrong with me was a slight cold.' Said

I: 'What a fool the man must have been!' Said the patient: 'Why, doctor, it was *you;* don't you remember it?' I thought for some time, and had to confess that now he mentioned it, I did have some vague, faint recollection of the occasion. Certainly he was not the only patient I had visited on a bicycle in the snow.

I did not at that time appreciate that the compulsive force in me that led me to get on with the job with a total disregard for my leisure, comfort and often for my meals, and the condition of mental strain, however unconsciously and habitually endured, which accompanied it, may have had a good deal to do with my occasional attacks of acute trigeminal neuralgia. Perhaps this self-disregarding attitude to my work was in itself some sort of a neurosis, though I was not aware of any masochism. There was a large element of identification with a suffering person, with those in distress. Such a one had sent to me for help and I must rescue him instantly.

The work of general practice was to me anything but a dull routine. There were, of course, the chronic patients, both in the surgery and for regular visits. There was that old lady of ninety-four up the road, who was bedridden and totally blind. At the request of her daughter, one visited her regularly once a week, on the same day at the same time, and sat by her bedside, holding her hand, and saying cheerful, kind words; then one probably put a stethescope on her heart and the base of her lungs. The daughter's case was of passing psychological interest. She complained that when at her office in the city, she was periodically getting hunches that her aged mother, left alone in bed for several hours, had taken a turn for the worst. In consequence, she had to go running home . . . only to find that the old lady was the same as usual. These fruitless journeys were on the increase. I then learnt that thirty odd years ago, when the daughter had been a young woman and the mother was about sixty, the daughter was engaged to be married. She had, however, told her fiancé that she could hardly marry him and abandon the blind and infirm, ageing lady. The impression was that the mother's infirmities, even at that time, would lead to an early demise, so the daughter had agreed to marry when mother had departed this life. Years had become decades, mother was still there, and the marriage still deferred. Finally, the man had married another; but the daughter still had her ageing mother. Her anticipation of happiness had depended upon the mother's death, and she had repressed her death wishes for quite a long time. It was not that she consciously wished her mother to be dead; on the contrary, every day she panicked lest her mother should die. Shall we leave it at that?

I can still remember the spotlessly clean sheets and other obvious signs of the assiduous care with which the old lady was nursed and looked after. All seemed to me to be the result of an over-compensation (against repressed death wishes), and this over-compensation was no doubt responsible for the prolongation of the old lady's frustrating life. Certainly it was not for me to interfere by any psychological interpretation or suggestion. No doubt there was or had been a great deal of love also. Mothers have tended their babies and children with equal assiduous care throughout the most troublesome and helpless years. It may be easy for them as it has an instinct basis, common to all mammals and even to birds. Should we deny merit on that account, and reserve it for what? For conditioned reflexes? Have acquired 'reflexes' more 'merit' than inherited ones? Perhaps there is nothing really adequate that a younger generation can do to repay loving and self-sacrificing parents for their devotion; nothing adequate they can do to mitigate the tragedy of nature's cruel 'repayment': increasing infirmity and final execution.

It was not only commonplace phenomena, such as this, encountered dozens of times a day in the course of a general practice, that gave one food for thought and for philosophical reflection; there were millions of things all the time. But the practically-minded practitioner, having to do his job as expeditiously as possible and having to get on to the next job, and above all having to make ends meet, to earn a living, and if possible to achieve a freedom from anxiety and the thrill of making more than a living, may be excused if he has little or no time for philosophy.

CHAPTER XI

PSYCHOGENESIS

ONE of the interesting aspects of work in this practice was the fairly frequent attendance at the local cottage hospital, where a surgeon by the name of Mr. Simmons used to perform almost every variety of operation. Surgical work had never been very congenial to me, and I fancy had grown less so, therefore I usually fell into the role of anaesthetist, while the particular practitioner who had sent the patient acted as Mr. Simmons' chief assistant. I gradually became increasingly interested in the very large proportion of perfectly normal appendices that were removed in this cottage hospital. It was not always easy to obtain possession of them after the operation—one was afraid of offending the susceptibilities of one's colleagues—but I always lent over and took a very careful look, and flattered myself that I could detect normality in an appendix from its outside appearance without having to dissect it. Now I come to think of it, I cannot remember more than one or two inflamed or abnormal appendices, though I remember dozens, it seems to me, of perfectly normal, pink, healthy ones. I began to wonder whether patients and doctors alike were, without knowing it, flogging this diagnostic horse or putting all their troubles and perplexities into this familiar and convenient form. Although I had not officially done any real psychological work, I got a hunch that many of these young people, knowing about appendicitis, somehow managed to divert their mental, emotional stresses and strains into this idea, managed to feel the pain physically, and successfully to suggest the reality of it all to their practitioner. What other explanation could there be for the removal of all these normal appendices?

Later on, amongst the mass of neurotic people, obviously the greater part of one's practice, who presented themselves at my surgery, came a pale, tall young woman who complained of a pain in her back, somewhere between her shoulder blades. Movement was completely unimpeded, there was no local rigidity, and I could find no cause whatsoever for the pain. I did think she was the sort of girl who ought to have a boy friend, but who was probably too shy and timid to ensnare one. She kept on attending, once or twice a week. The pain was evidently not always in the same place, and then after a week or so's absence, she appeared complaining of a pain in her abdomen. I almost watched this settle down into an appendix pain, but I had been forewarned and was convinced that this girl did not have appendicitis, acute or otherwise. However, I could neither cure her completely nor get rid of her. She kept on coming to me, at least once a week or once a fortnight, and getting a bottle of medicine. She seemed to me a little anaemic, but otherwise healthy enough. Nearly always there was this vague abdominal trouble, with discomfort about the appendix region. Many times I examined her, and found equivalent tenderness wherever I cared to put a little pressure. However, for one reason or another I was convinced that it was just *her*, and that nobody could do anything about it.

However, after she had been coming to me on and off for something like two years, suddenly all her family got very excited about her. She was a good-class girl. Her mother interviewed me, her father interviewed me, everybody interviewed me. They all wanted to know what I was doing about their Alice; she could not go on like this, complaining on and off. She had been attending for nearly two years, and if I could not cure her, why didn't I send her to somebody else. Well, I did. I arranged a consultation with my great surgeon friend in Harley Street. I can still remember it pretty clearly, and my having to put off all my busy practice work in order to dance attendance on the great man, but I was not sorry to do so because I was genuinely puzzled about this girl. I remember his taking a detailed history, and I remember his examining her, poking his fingers deep into her right iliac fossa over Mc-Burney's point, and her complaining bitterly of its extreme tenderness. I remember, too, that it seemed to me she did not react violently enough, considering the depth of his pressure at that moment.

After the examination, the surgeon took me into an adjoining room and said to me very seriously: 'My boy, you have been "cooking" a chronic appendix for two years.' Well, there it was. We took her into a nursing home, and at his request, I assisted at the operation. And what did we take out? A perfectly normal appendix! He was so incredulous that he actually enlarged his operation incision (it was a median one) and carefully, with his gloved hand, examined, by direct contact, every organ in her abdomen. He felt her kindeys, the pelves and ureters, he felt her gall bladder and its ducts, he actually squeezed her gall bladder and emptied it to make quite sure it had no stones or concretions in it. Presently he went down into her pelvis and carefully examined each ovary between his fingers; he felt her fallopian tubes and uterus. Finally, he had to admit that there definitely was no organic disease whatsoever in her abdomen or pelvis. We stitched her up, this alabaster-like, attractive girl, now with a long, red, vertical scar up the centre of her abdomen. The surgeon carefully warned the matron, sisters and nurses that nobody must on any account let the patient know that her appendix was normal. Like most surgeons, his psychotherapy was limited to the employment of powerful suggestion. His theory was that she, having concentrated all her troubles into the conviction of diseased appendix, if she now knew that the 'diseased' appendix had been completely removed, the result would be that all her troubles would be completely removed! I smiled a little inwardly, but my first impression later was that perhaps he was right, not in his surgery, but in his psychotherapy, and I was wrong.

The thing I shall never forget is the look on the face of that young woman when I visited her in the nursing home the following morning. Her expression was rapt. She looked ecstatic; one might almost say, as though she had at last come into the Kingdom of Heaven and seen God.

> ' . . . the wonder was not yet quite gone
> From that still look of hers. . . .'

I stared at her calm, serene expression; I had never seen anything like it on her face before throughout those two years. What could this mean? Admittedly she had achieved her two-year-long objective and had her appendix removed. But why such ecstasy?

I am convinced that the psychopathology of the whole thing was this: What her libido had really needed was normal treatment from a normal man; that is to say, love, sex and orgasm. But such wants, or such wants in that form, were inadmissible to her consciousness; besides, she would not have had the courage, or even the social

courage, to find a man. What could the poor girl do? Illness was all
around her, her mother frequently went to the doctor, and illness
was admissible. There was no moral censorship of that. Indeed,
religion taught, or could be interpreted as teaching, that whereas
to seek the gratification of one's lusts was wicked, suffering, to
suffer the crucifixion of the flesh, was a virtue. Thus, by a maso-
chistic perversion of instinct gratification, both it and the superego
(conscience) could be satisfied by the same symptom. It all started
in her back, a fact which I had not forgotten, and which had therefore prejudiced me against the subsequent suggestion of appendicitis.
(I fancy that a larger proportion of back troubles than of any other
localised symptom, are psychogenic, in spite of the latest fashion of
slipped-disc diagnosis, unheard of in my young days.) This girl
having been to me, seen me and taken courage, the pains had shifted
nearer the appropriate region. The concept of appendicitis was
offered by all the rules of medicine. What she wanted for her 'pain'
her unconcious knew all right, but her conscious level was prevented by censorship from knowing. It was altered, and symboli-
cally represented by a knife, by a mechanism comparable to that
which had displaced her discomfort from genital to abdomen. For
two years she had longed for this 'knife', perhaps loosely associated
with me. Now, at last, thanks to the great surgeon, she had had
the knife; it had entered her; the libidinal wish had been realised;
life was wonderful!

I have seen comparable expressions of quiet satisfaction, a form
of ecstasy, on the faces of so many mothers just after their child
has been born. What a pity it is that we are all so silly! I remembered the succession of patients, nearly all or all, as far as my
memory goes, whom I had seen having their normal appendices removed in that cottage hospital. Is this the price of 'civilisation', of
the censorship? Is it this censorship of nature that produces unnatural manifestations, perversions, neuroses, illnesses . . . and
operations? Recently a patient under analysis said to me: 'My conflict is between heart and head. But isn't that what civilisation
means—being split in half for the benefit of one's neighbours?'

I would not like to suggest that the only interest in a general
practice is psychological. I dare say there are many practitioners,
past and present, who, if one asked them to give a representative
sample of their patients, would think exclusively of those who had

organic diseases, and might find it hard at first to remember many of those who had not. In my own case, at the moment, the reverse seems to be true. I can remember dozens, hundreds of patients with psychogenic disorders and illnesses, and find it a little difficult to recall many of those, and there must have been many, who had organic diseases in which the psychogenic factors were, or at first sight appeared to be, relatively negligible. Perhaps experience and investigation has made me a little biased. I was certainly not biased in favour of the psychogenesis of human ills when I first entered general practice. On the contrary; I can still remember how I used to spend enormous quantities of time examining a complainer from head to toe, with every possible diagnostic device, to find the alleged organic source of his or her complaint. I used to go through all the cranial nerves; in some instances, I used extraordinary instruments, which I carried about with me, and took drops of people's blood to find the colour index. I used to look at their optic nerves with an ophthalmoscope, test their reflexes, touch, pain, hot and cold, stethoscope all over their chests, front and back, blood pressures; and I acquired a sensitiveness with my fingers to the feel of almost everything in the relaxed abdomen. I was very slow to learn that not one in a hundred of these people showed or possessed any appreciable organic disease. It was said of me in the neighbourhood that 'one thing you can be certain of, if you go to that doctor, is the most thorough examination you have ever had in your life.' I was as rabid a fool, or innocent, as Saint Paul—before his conversion.

It took experience to 'bias' me in favour of psychogenesis. I certainly came from my hospital-training with a bias the other way. In general practice, however, I learnt that even such patently physical things as cut hands (not to speak of cut throats) usually had a psychogenic factor which was commonly the essential cause. This applied also to most accidents, whether to oneself or to others. I remember the occasion when Mrs. Lilley dashed through the waiting-room into my surgery, sobbing, with the terrible news that her small infant had scalded itself with a pail of boiling water. No, she did not want me to run round, it had been rushed off to hospital, but she did not know what to do, she had come to me, could I do something for her nerves? I ran into the dispensary and said aloud, more to myself than to my experienced dispenser: 'I want some-

thing sedative for a woman whose baby has just scalded itself with a
pail of boiling water.' She, knowing the character of most of my
clientele, remarked quite confidently: 'That will be Mrs. Lilley's
baby.' I said: 'You're right, but how did you know?' She said:
'Well, Mrs. Lilley is the only mother I can think of to whom such a
thing would happen.' This gave me a moment's food for thought.
Were even such accidents due directly or indirectly to the psychology of the person, or at least were the dice of life's hazards
psychogenically weighted?

I remember, too, a young woman who came to me with early
tuberculosis. She had recently given birth to a baby; she was very
young, nineteen, and had only a year ago married a lad of eighteen,
and had been taken off to live in his mother's house. The mother
had given them the 'top flat' to live in; it was an attic with one tiny
window. Yes, she had lived in it for a whole year, but her husband
was only occasionally in it; just at nights. He spent his evenings
downstairs in the lounge with his mother and other members of his
family, sitting by the fire. She was not allowed in the lounge, nor
apparently in any other part of the house. He commonly had his
meals with them; she was supposed to look after herself. She often
neglected her meals, could not be bothered. Yes, she had gone
through her pregnancy in that attic; and now she had early tuberculosis of lung. Well, I did not know, but the possibility occurred to
me that in addition to the physical effects of pregnancy, the general
psychological situation, including depression and its physical
accompaniments or consequences, may have had something to do
with the initiation of her decline. It would not be surprising if some
mothers, who are emotionally married to their son, wished, unconsciously at least, for the death of their successful rival. Unconscious wishes can and do achieve not only the production of dreams,
but also the implementation and execution of them in the real
world—often unwittingly. Evidence? Well, there is the evidence of
the continuation of life, propagated by instincts which are not
necessarily conscious; remember, beetles do it too.

One of the minor disadvantages of professional work is the little
trickle of women, some of them very young girls, who present
themselves with unwanted pregnancies. One feels sometimes that
there ought to be a panel of benevolent and unbiased jurists em-
powered to treat each such case according to its individual merits,

taking into consideration the expediency of the situation. Either
that, or illegitimate childbirth should be as triumphantly applauded
socially as legitimate. To my mind, there is no sense in torturing
human beings just because they have lived in accordance with
nature's edict and with relative disregard for the artificial and unnatural rules of society, too much, in my opinion, initiated and
influenced by an outworn religious sadism. However, it fortunately
turned out that many of these pregnancies were pseudo-preg-
nancies, purely psychogenic in origin due to a combination of the
body's unconscious insistence on being pregnant and the mind's
acute fear, guilt and anxiety on a conscious plane. What the mind
fears is commonly the age-long compulsions (instincts) of its own
body, which, fortunately for its survival, have the power to over-
whelm this puny newcomer (conscious ideas and moralities) in the
field of nature.

Many of these cases turned out this way, but not all. I can remember two pretty young sisters whom I first visited when they
were both in the same double bed together, suffering from measles.
The younger one, a particularly nice girl of, I think, less than
seventeen, was later brought to me by her mother, the latter in a
frantic state of distress, for a three or four months old pregnancy,
incurred, she said, when the girl had been sent with her sister for a
holiday on a farm, the responsible male being a lad of sixteen. The
mother recognised that nothing could be done about it. She had
approached the boy's mother, who proved to be a horrid woman.
Nevertheless, they managed eventually to get a court order for ten
shillings a week. As one can imagine, there was a great disturbance
throughout the family; but subsequently this girl had a perfectly
healthy and delightful baby. The whole neighbourhood knew
everything about it, and remembering the distress and tears, it was
amusing to see the infant's grandmother experiencing a new lease
of life by virtue of wheeling the infant about in a pram and proudly
exhibiting it to everybody. I was at the practice long enough to
see the young mother subsequently married to a very nice man and
to attend her for another baby.

Perhaps it is the unrepresentative incidents in general practice
which, on that very account, impress themselves most on one's
memory. The daily routine included, of course, a large proportion
of commonplace things. Severe organic diseases, medical and sur-

gical, are usually passed on for hospital treatment. They are the
exception not the rule. The practitioner is left with a host of minor
ills, and an overwhelming proportion of psychogenic distresses,
with or without physical symptoms. It was easy to verify this impression by looking at one's panel cards, some thousands strong.
About four cases in five had never once presented themselves to
their doctor. Of the remaining one in five, the majority had attended
once or twice, or maybe three times. At the other end of
the scale, a small proportion of the thousands, numbering perhaps a
few hundred people in all, were continually popping in. Some of
them, it seemed, could not live without a twice-a-week visit to the
doctor. Was it right to say they never really had anything the
matter with them, or that they always had something the matter
with them, something apparently incurable?

I have heard that comparable statistics arose out of a war-time
investigation of accidents in minor munition factories. It was found
that nineteen out of twenty of the employees had never had an
accident throughout several years. Of the remaining five per cent,
a few had had one or two accidents; but ninety-odd per cent of all
the accidents that had happened in these factories were shared
between a handful of people, most of whom had each had dozens.
They were called the accident-prone group, and it was considered
best to give them work which did not endanger themselves or
others. Thus it is seen that even statistics alone, without any
knowledge of psychology and without any theories of psychopathology, can be held to establish the psychogenesis not only of illnesses but even of a proneness to accidents.

It is not only the suicide whose 'mental balance is disturbed', the
unconscious mind can harbour, at the same time, the antithetical
impulses of destruction, self-destruction, construction and self-
preservation; and express these simultaneously, in various proportions, by both internal (bodily) and external activities; all
without the co-operation, or even the knowledge, of the conscious
ego. It is from such unconscious behaviour that we get, short of
death or suicide, internal disturbances, called illnesses, and external disturbances called accidents.

There are cases that occur in general practice where it is almost
impossible to avoid coupling the outward behaviour of a person,
such as his sexual behaviour towards a mate, with the inward be-

haviour of his organs—for instance his heart, proverbially susceptible, and even his stomach and intestines—that immediately ensues when he is suddenly deprived of this external situation. It is as though the activities which were previously being expressed *outwardly*, for instance sexually, continue, when the external situation is brought to an end, *internally*, with just as much energy and violence. Hence a quiescent or allegedly healed duodenal ulcer is re-activated, and a sudden abdominal crisis, such as perforation ensues. Instances of this nature were gradually accumulating and coming more and more to my notice in regard to almost every alleged and real organic illness. Pseudo-cancer, psuedo-cyesis (a condition in which all the symptoms of pregnancy, including absence of menstruation, are displayed without there being any pregnancy present) rheumatism, gastric and duodenal ulcers, colitis, and probably any and every variety of organic illness, not excluding tuberculosis, were all becoming more clearly seen by me to have an initiating, or at least a precipitating, factor in the mind.

I remember meeting the late Dr. Morton, who was then Medical Officer, and I believe at one time Governor, of Holloway Prison in North London. He told me some fascinating stories about the self-mutilating activities of prisoners. He told me of alleged criminals who swallowed safety pins and nails, and lots of them who mutilated themselves with knives and other instruments. It was not without interest that a favourite region for mutilation amongst males of this sort was that of their genitals. He instances a case where a man had actually cut open his scrotum and removed his testicles. While listening to him, I felt that the psychology of these people, obviously people with a psychotic (insane) streak, a streak which no doubt accounted for their criminality as well as their self-injury, had something in common with the psychology of a large proportion of my clientele who were constantly 'achieving' accidents and minor illnesses. The people who kept coming in to see me twice a week or so with colds, bronchitis, 'flu, gastric and intestinal disturbances and so on, were, though unconsciously, putting themselves in the way of these illnesses, just as Dr. Morton's cases put themselves in the way of arrest and punishment, as well as self-inflicted injuries. The need to receive punishment, even in the form of illness, may be just as compulsive as the need to inflict punishment. The difference depends upon the direction which the compulsion takes, upon whether we have our 'knife' in others or in ourselves. The former is more usual and more normal.

Nevertheless, it was not possible to be quite sure as to how much of this tendency to minor illness was acquired by the individual, and how much of it might have been due to an inherited tendency. No doubt some of us are less fortunate in having inherited a less robust physical, as well as mental, constitution than others; the fault may lie in the egg. With a wider view, we may say that every individual is a combination of what he inherits from the egg, together with the action upon him of the environment which he encounters, and the reaction by his nature upon that environment. Thus, psychology and science would explode the idea of responsibility, except in a very superficial sense. This does not mean that society should abandon the principle of protecting itself. A mosquito may not be responsible for its proclivity to sting us, but we do not therefore feel constrained to preserve its life.

I was becoming more and more impressed with the fact that, while the practitioner confines his attentions to such things as the bit of phlegm in his patient's bronchi, he is ignoring the important issue that that phlegm, and everything else internal and external that happens to that patient, is commonly connected with his emotional mental attitudes, connected with emotional patterns which formed in him at an early age of his infancy and childhood, patterns whose connection with the outside world was, in the first place, at a time when his outside world was more or less limited to his parents. Psychological evidence is constantly showing us that *we go through life repeating these early patterns, and manipulating our environment to facilitate our repetition of them.* To what pattern did all these recurrent and chronic illnesses belong? It seemed that an element might well be some level of infantile unhappiness. The deepest level, in this respect, apart from inheritance, is that connected with the gratification and frustration of instinctual needs. The baby that is left to 'cry it out' in his pram is already at a preparatory school which will qualify him to sit twice weekly in the general practitioner's surgery.

These further investigations are probably the fruit of subsequent research and investigation. At that time, I was daily occupied with my very busy general practice. All I can say is that impressions of this nature began to force themselves upon my mind. I remembered the dispenser's remark: 'That would be Mrs. Lilley's baby that got scalded.' I am reminded now that this particular woman had three children, each of whom met with a fatal accident in infancy, though in one case the 'fatal accident' took the form of pneumonia. Ungenerously, I suspect that this too was the result of some mental quality or lack of quality in that particular mother. These other people who kept on seeing me, and having their bottle of medicine so regularly that if they were away for two or three weeks one would wonder that had happened to them, doubtless needed something or somebody, though in so far as the somebody was the doctor and the something the magical bottle of medicine, they must have been both right and wrong. Evidence that they were wrong lay in the fact that they showed no sign of ever getting well and requiring no further attention, and evidence that they were right was suggested by their finding sufficient relief or consolation to cause them to come back again for more.

I was beginning to feel that the whole of this subject of medicine, and for that matter of surgery too, was taking a somewhat short-sighted view of the causes and nature of human troubles. It was concentrating exclusively upon the end-products, the results or sequelae, and that was no way to get at the root of a thing, or to cure it, or indeed to do anything very useful about it in a big way. It became more and more clear to me that the roots and beginnings of practically all these things lay in something less palpable, less see-able, less discoverable, than the body and its organs. When we asked the old question: 'How did Mr. Baldwin get to the House of Commons?' we did not like the answer in terms of the physical structure and physiology of his leg muscles. Were we doing something of that nature in our medical and surgical questions and answers? If any of us moves a limb or a muscle, the phenomenon of the movement itself is not the matter of primary importance or interest; the limb does not move on its own account. What is important is that there was a thought, something in the mind, which initiated or led to that physical movement. Similarly, if an organ moves from healthy function to diseased function, or for that matter from rest to any function, there is, generally speaking, a movement in the mind, in the unconscious if not in the conscious mind, which initiated the movement or the change.

What about all these patients? I was growing tired of studying end-products, whether they were those of muscular movement, of skin rashes, or of visceral movement and change. How wonderful it would be if we could discover how these things really started, what started them! And here were all my patients, or at least the majority of my patients, each offering me a clue to the investigation of this infinitely more important human problem.

In short, I was beginning to recognise that I had studied the wrong subject, that what initiated people's illnesses was, generally speaking, not that some individual organ took it into its head, as it were, to go wrong ; but that the larger question of successful and happy adjustment to environment, adjustment that ensured the absence of anxiety and the necessary gratification of instinct, was at the basis of the whole thing.

By this devious route, by this enthusiastic interest, first in natural science and subsequently in medicine and surgery, particularly in the light of my general practice experience, I had been led back to my original line of enquiry. Can the riddle of the universe be divided into compartments? Anyhow, I felt I would prefer to study wider aspects of it than this branch, physical, organic disorder and disease, end-products, a branch which I had already decided could not lead me directly to the source of the trouble or solve more than a very small fraction of the riddle, the riddle which I was beginning to see was really all-embracing and indivisible.

At these surgeries, when a woman came in and remarked, as occasionally happened: 'Doctor, I think I have cancer,' I used promptly to write down on the case paper 'Anxiety Neurosis', without looking up. With my ripening experience, I felt little inclination to examine her or even to look at the alleged trouble. I knew that hers was simply a case of anxiety and nothing more; and it always was. Nevertheless, one had, of course, to listen to the story and to do the expected examination. I cannot remember one instance in which it altered the immediate diagnosis.

Presently, there was nothing for it but to investigate why this particular person was suffering from this anxiety. The answer did not usually lie in anything she could tell you on a conscious plane. Alleged causes or sources of the anxiety were of a piece with her supposition that she had cancer. They were practically always secondary products of the anxiety, some idea on to which she pinned the anxiety which was already present. Again and again in the case of such patients, one found that either they were orgastically frigid, or suffering from some degree of psychosexual frigidity, or that their husbands were impotent, too quick, or otherwise sexually inadequate, or sexually negligent of them on account of another attachment, or just disinterested. The woman would commonly say: 'But, doctor, that sort of thing doesn't interest me at all.' Then one would find that there had been a time, perhaps in her courtship days or until the birth of her first child, when it had interested her very much; often she had been far from frigid at some earlier period of her life. Commonly the sequence of events was this: In order to avoid further pregnancies, the husband had taken to practising withdrawal, *coitus interruptus*. The consequence of this had been that gradually and imperceptibly her interest in his sexual approaches had lessened until it had disappeared altogether; thus she could say quite truthfully: 'That sort of thing doesn't interest me at all.' It did not; but it was only a matter of *how long* between this acquired disinterestedness and frigidity to the outcrop of a host of anxiety symptoms. When they reached the dimensions of 'cancer', she presented herself to the doctor.

Anxiety in young people was commonly a sequel to love-making which entailed stimulation but not full gratification. Even abstinence, in the case of a maturing and alive instinct, repressed or otherwise, could cause this condition. Thus I discovered from my own clinical experience that these states of anxiety were connected with factors in the person's life which he or she was completely disregarding. The patients rarely had a clue as to why they were in this uncomfortable, nervous condition. On the contrary, they usually found an alleged cause, a hypochondriacal 'cause', to attach to it. The forms of interference with natural function were legion, and affected different people with degrees of strain proportionate to their *constitutional* ability to tolerate frustration and to hold tension. I was gradually forced to the conclusion that a lot of my cases of minor illnesses were initiated by and founded upon causes of this nature. Later I grew to recognise that such factors, that is to say factors in the current sexual life of the patient, whether overt or intrapsychic, were often nothing more than a precipitating cause, a sort of spearhead of the neurosis. More deeply hidden psychopathological conditions were commonly the soil upon which these current disturbances grew. Among these underlying factors, an apparently constant one appeared to be the *emotional condition during infancy.*

A lot of these people, though not all, had gone through some degree of neurotic disturbance in early life. Many had definitely had symptoms, such as fears, phobias, tantrums, or even fits, and functional abnormalities such as bedwetting. This last habit was often protracted to a comparatively late age in childhood. One might say that practically all these 'infantile neuroses' are common in everybody's childhood to a certain extent or to a certain degree. The difference in the case of people suffering from neuroses and their sequelae (illnesses) was essentially a difference in degree rather than in kind. Even then, it seemed that the condition might not in adult life have become active, or so active, had it not been for the additional strain caused by *current precipitating factors.* Looking back into childhood like this, it was becoming obvious to me that the problem was a very deep and complicated one. It was one thing to see something of its nature in the present day, to diagnose it, and quite another thing to discover its causes, particularly the remote or early factors involved.

A disappointing element here was that if one took the trouble to unravel the patients' family history, that of their parents and other relatives, one commonly discovered a host of similar tendencies in them also, sometimes identical in their symptomatology, though frequently presenting themselves in a different form. It appeared that all forms of neurosis were related one to another, and that the causative factors often extended far into the past, far beyond the individual's lifetime. However, it seemed to me that the manifestations of these conditions were so diffuse, diverse and all-embracing that the subject was one more worth studying than were the occasional end-products of these emotional states, end-products which were the subject matter of the medical studies which I had been taught. The whole subject extended beyond medicine; there were all sorts of eccentricities, and peculiarities and minor abnormalities: the people who were full of dietetic fads, the people who were addicted to treatment by osteopaths, the physical-medicine addicts, the patent-medicine addicts, and for that matter the bottle-of-medicine addicts, those to whom I, in my general practitioner-capacity, was assigned.

I have made earlier some reference to the statistics of accident-prone people. It seemed to me that my work was mostly confined to illness-prone people. It seemed that some of these people had only to take off an overcoat to catch a cold; but what was of interest was that their proneness to minor illnesses varied in accordance with their emotional state at the particular time. They needed something. I began to think that a lot of them really needed a suitable mate. On account of the nature of our civilisation, our moral code, and our acceptance of medicine and doctors as a perfectly legitimate part of it, the poor things commonly thought that what they needed was a doctor. Was one to subscribe indefinitely to this neurotic or psychotic set-up of civilisation, or would it not be more worthy of one's intelligence to investigate?

With such thoughts in my mind, back to me came the appendix case I have previously described at some length; the young woman who looked so ecstatically sublime the morning after her operation, as though she had achieved her soul's and body's desire, like a woman should look the morning after her bridal night—but rarely does. Well, she came back, and what did she complain of? The identical pain in the identical place! She said to me: 'Doctor, it must be adhesions after the operation. Somebody told me it might be.' But I had had enough of this. I had known all along that one gratification, however large and devastating, could not gratify the libido permanently. It would have been easy for me at that stage to have talked to her too frankly and openly. I could have said: 'You have come back to me, but I am not going to gratify you. When you achieve gratification, you will need it again and again, if it proves to be any good, and heaven knows, with all this displacement of it on to medical and surgical ideas, attempts to get it back into normal channels may fail.' However, I felt it was no part of my duty to subscribe to or to encourage this displacement-tendency which I had now come to regard as a sort of accepted and permitted 'perversion'.

But if that was to be my attitude, what was I doing in general practice, where an acceptance of this principle, the principle that I was now calling a perversion, was the essence of one's work and the source of one's income? In any case, I was getting a bit tired of what I frivolously described as running round the streets and putting my hands on people's stomachs. Palpating these bellies

might be good fun in many ways; one obtained an interesting bit
of insight into people's minds, and after all, possibly accentuated by
my anatomical and physiological studies, I was not at all averse to
their bodies; in fact, I think I liked bodies, they were interesting,
like mine. Nevertheless, that was not sufficient excuse or justification for spending my life with this amusement. What I wanted to
do, what I must do, what I intended to do, was to investigate the
nature of the mind which lay behind it all. In addition, I may say
that I had reached a stage when no other course was possible. For
instance, when this appendicectomy-young-lady came back to
me, I found myself asking her questions about her background, even
about her infancy, her relationship to her mother and father, and
so on. In due course, she began to talk to me spontaneously, of her
own accord; the story of her childhood unfolded itself, and presently
she took to unburdening her heart. Curiously enough, in a way that
I could not quite measure, it so came about that something was
loosened up in her. She actually began to take a little interest in a
male acquaintance or hanger-on, whom she had not, up to that
time, so much as noticed. In due course, she began to tell me about
it; of course, I encouraged it for all I was worth. It took me a little
time to realise that, while she was using me as her confidant, I
was, and for that matter always had been, more important to her
emotionally than was anybody else, I hoped it was not more than
anyone else could become. The problem became two-fold: not only
how to get her normally interested in a male friend, but, what
seemed even more difficult, how to get her disinterested in me,
how to cure her evident compulsion to keep visiting my surgery in
order to tell me, now not exclusively about her abdominal pain,
but about everything. I began to see that the subject to which my
interest was turning had several aspects. There was the research
aspect, and there was also, in the meantime, the immediate practical
aspect, the question of a technique which might enable one to put
people on their own feet, and to help them to make their
own healthy and health-giving adjustments to others, and at
the same time to free them from the need to keep everlastingly
leaning their whole weight on me. Was it possible that
a method could be devised to cope with all this? Well, science
had always been faced with difficulties in its investigation
into the unknown, and surely the difficulties of this peculiar

new psychological science were not necessarily more insurmountable than the difficulties which faced the first physicists and
chemists.

I mentioned something of my psychological problem, with re-
reference to a particular case, to old Dr. Fisher, whom I now very
rarely had any occasion to meet. He said: 'Yes, of course, the practice is full of them; every practice is, but you don't want to worry
about that. They are the mainstay of the practice, and fortunately
they cause you no anxiety. Yes, of course they get attached to you,
that is what keeps a practice going; where would any doctor be
without his hosts of neurotic patients with their minor illnesses?
It is only through them that you are kept in a position to deal
with the real illnesses when they arise, the people we send to
hospital.'

Then it came out that he occasionally sent a selected case to a
particular eminent analyst. He told me about one of these. I was
amazed to learn that the patient got better. 'How on earth,' said I
'could anybody cure a thing like that?' I had learnt and understood
enough about it to recognise the extraordinary difficulties in the
way of a cure. It interests me now to reflect that the Tavistock
Clinic, at which I subsequently worked for about seventeen years,
finally altered the printed word 'Cure', which had long been on its
summary case-sheet for statistical purposes, to the word
'Amelioration'.

I reflected that life itself is doubtless synonymous with all
sorts of mental imperfections, imperfect adjustments to reality, to
environment, to family, to people, to the civilisation in which we
live, to the laws, to other nations—all based, I have since discovered, upon intrapsychic conflict, mostly unconscious. Life is
synonymous with attempts to achieve better and better adjustments, with attempts to achieve amelioration; but cure! that is
only a phantasy, a phantasy from which has arisen the concept of
paradise.

In those days, however much of a philosopher I may have been or
have aspired to be, I was nothing if I was not practical. No doubt
the practice of medicine, particularly in general practice, would
make even a poet practical. In the back of my mind, if not in the
front, I was becoming more and more concerned with the problem
of how to give myself time and opportunity to study this new aspect

of medicine, and of everything else that had been forced upon my attention, while at the same time ensuring that my income remained adequate to provide me with the wherewithal for study and research.

CHAPTER XII

ANALYSIS

AFTER I had been two or three years on my own a colleague of mine, more recently qualified, asked me if I could find room for him in my now flourishing practice. Was this the ram caught in the thicket? He was a nice, quiet sort of chap, and I thought he would do fairly well, for I was, by this time, quite sure that some change in the routine of my life was due. It was obvious to me that it was not going to be good enough to continue using up every moment of, my available time, putting my hand on a succession of abdomens all day long, as I described it, and merely having what was left of the day or night after ten p.m. for reading or recreation. There was no possibility of fitting the study of my new enthusiasm, psychology, into this routine. Space had to be made for it.

I could not afford to have an assistant, but I arranged a very satisfactory partnership agreement with Dr. Saunderson, which had the advantage of releasing me during the latter half of the day. This enabled me to attend lectures and courses of study in the afternoon. This freedom was very exhilarating, because I knew exactly what I wanted to do with it. I was free to study this new-found, intriguing subject, and I was contemplating a way to set about doing this in a systematic manner.

The diligent reading of Freud's immense classic, *The Interpretation of Dreams* set me back a bit, though fortunately it did not put me off altogether; however, the attendance of a short, two to three week course in Psychotherapy for Practitioners, at the Tavistock Clinic, revived my interest with added enthusiasm—and perhaps unwarranted optimism. I attended the ordinary psychology syllabus at University College, where I was fortunate enough to encounter a lecturer, Dr. J. C. Flugel, whose interests were wider than those of laboratory experimental psychology. He took the opportunity provided by his series of lectures to teach us something of the unconscious, and the simpler concepts of psychoanalysis. All this, in the light of my clinical experiences in general practice, I found most intriguing. What I was really waiting for, however, was the orthodox, academic course of study in psychiatry, designed for the Diploma in Psychological Medicine; not that I aspired to taking that or any other diploma; I simply thought it would be a study relevant to my interest, the mystery of illness and of everything else. There were two places at which the course was conducted: at Maudsley Hospital, and at Bethlem Royal Hospital, then in Lambeth. I chose Bethlem because it was nearer. The course was exacting and of the crammer variety. It involved being in the lecture-room at two p.m. and continuing, practically without getting up, till six-thirty p.m. Very soon I was plunged into a life in some respects as strenuous as that from which I had freed myself. I found that with the morning surgery, which I still conducted, in North London and my list of visits, I had a scramble to get finished by one-thirty. I would then jump into the tube train, and travel down to North Lambeth station. Lunch was out of the question, so I carried a small attaché case in which I had several bananas, as this proved the simplest and quickest way of taking a mid-day meal. The tube was always deserted at that time of day, and I had no difficulty in eating from my attaché case without embarrassment. I would arrive just in time for the two o'clock lecture. There was another lecture at three o'clock, half an hour for tea, a lecture from four-thirty to five-thirty, and again from five-thirty to six-thirty; a very packed afternoon, as each subject was entirely different from the preceding one, and nothing was ever repeated. It was very like my first year at St. Thomas's Medical School all over again. The subjects included lectures from the professor of anatomy, confined to the central nervous system, every detail of its structure, including histological (microscopic) examination, and a full course of lectures in neurology; this, in addition to the expected normal and abnormal psychology, psychiatry, mental deficiency, pathology and laboratory work. Everything was very concentrated and crammed together. To supplement lectures, evenings were commonly spent staining slides of the nervous system in the path. lab.; and, at least twice a week, sitting for hours in a private room with a succession of selected mental patients.

I cannot describe how much I enjoyed every minute of this work. It may seem rather extraordinary that this should be so; I was, as it were, back at school, or the equivalent of the medical school, absorbing information about new subjects, and yet every fibre of me knew that it was absolutely my milieu. Why had I put it off all these years, while I wasted time in the Army in India (though perhaps the building of the telescope and the study of astronomy was not waste of time), and while I rushed around feeling people's stomachs all day? Thank heaven I had found my vocation again, I hoped before it was too late. I paused to wonder what peculiarity there could be about my particular psychological make-up that I was, even at an age over thirty, preferring the absorbing of new information to any other occupation. Was I temperamentally the perpetual student? Had I never grown up?

Culture and civilisation and the training we give the young tend to defer, to put off, the biological purpose of the individual's life for as long a period as possible. It is as though we think the longer we can prepare for living, the better we will be when we start to live. The individual is still physically and physiologically developed to begin reproductive life probably at fourteen or fifteen, and in tropical climates earlier, but it is usual for such matters not to be countenanced until the middle twenties or later. I have a good deal of evidence in support of my theory that it is the biologically and psychologically stressful years between puberty and marriage which are largely responsible for the strain put upon individuals that results in so large a proportion of them having their predisposition to subsequent neurosis aroused to breaking point. And here was I, a conspicuous product of this potentially harmful, cultural pressure, still unmarried and delighting in being a student again in the thirties.

It was wonderful studying in an advanced way and to an advanced degree these illuminating subjects. I did not resent very much the tedium of application to the anatomy and histology of the central nervous system. In spite of my previous experience at the medical school, I did not even now fully realise that these scientific studies, however intriguing and satisfying, would have no bearing upon the clinical problems which would subsequently present themselves. Perhaps I did not want to realise this. It would be wonderful if, knowing the pathway of fibres through the central nervous system, one could thereby, as it were, put one's finger on what this or that neurotic patient was suffering from, and even perhaps put it right. Again I was holding the wrong end of the stick, hoping it was the right end. However, it provided a wonderfully exhilarating and satisfying pastime . . . so long as one did not have to apply it in clinical practice. Maybe for most of the time I deluded myself that I was learning what I wanted to know, the mystery of the human mind. Did McDougall know it? He wrote with great confidence, as though he did. Well, it was easier and more comfortable to believe that he had at least *something* to teach.

It was not until I had been studying at Bethlem for quite a time that I found I could no longer escape the realisation that all these intriguing and interesting studies, including the greater part of psychiatry itself, were, to say the least of it, insufficiently illuminating when one was confronted with an actual psychotic patient, and was trying to understand the nature, mechanism and origin of his peculiarities. It was only after a considerable time that I realised that I had now absorbed perhaps all the essentials, everything that mattered, that these particular branches of science were able to teach, and yet I did not find that I had a sufficiently complete or satisfying knowledge of how the mind worked, and how normality, neurosis and psychosis came into being. My exhilarating anticipations were beginning to give place to a realisation that disappoinment lay in store for me if I continued exclusively along these well-trodden scientific paths. Anyhow, I knew of no other paths. Well, what was I to do with all this learning I had absorbed, and with which I had now got to a stage when it seemed to be offering me nothing more, nothing really new or sufficiently illuminating? I became so disappointed in it that I did not know what to do with it. It was in this spirit I finally decided that I might as well sit for the Diploma, like the others were doing.

When I began my interest in psychology, when I planned my psychological studies, when I got Saunderson to take over nearly all the general practice for me, when I began the strenuous life at Bethlem, and for a long time after, I had had no thought at any time of sitting for an examination in the subject. I had been motivated simply and solely by an interest, a desire to know, exactly parallel with my disinterested interest in philosophy. I had even had the idea of spending my life researching in the mind, to try and understand how it worked and what it was all about. This had nothing whatsoever to do with the examinations. Thus I have no hesitation in saying that my decision to sit for an examination in psychology was a sign to me not of success, but of failure. It was a mark of the stage of disappointment I had reached. One could do no better with all this stuff I had been taught, for so many months, than to sit for an exam. in it, and perhaps get some new letters after one's name. I even felt inclined to disdain the exam. However, everyone else was busy preparing to sit for it. The fifteen or sixteen people in the post-graduate class at Bethlem all had their minds rivetted upon the exam. as though that was all that mattered. I sent up my name in a very different spirit.

Much to my surprise, as I was fully aware that I had not as yet learnt what I had set out to learn, I found the papers easy, and was quite certain of the result long before it was published. In fact, this examination experience so surprised me (knowing my own real ignorance) that I even began to think: why not sit for the M.D. in Psychological Medicine? After all, I had only a M.B., B.S., and sooner or later in one's life it might be as well to transform this into an M.D. Of course, it might have been more usual or appropriate to sit for the M.D. in General Medicine, but here I was, studying all this D.P.M. work, which was at least a portion of the syllabus for the M.D. in Psychiatry, so wouldn't it be an opportunity to get this higher qualification without undue trouble? I spoke to the senior Medical Officer at Bethlem, who was one of our lecturers. He was scornful and scoff-ful. He said: 'But my dear chap, the M.D. in Psychiatry is an examination for specialists, people who have worked in mental hospitals for years and years, and who have specialised in the subject.' He rather implied that I was only a general practitioner who was somewhat crazily playing about with this, his subject. He practically said: 'Don't waste your time with such ideas, you haven't got an earthly.' Well, his attitude so annoyed me that I immediately sent up my application papers. I was three or four weeks late in applying, after the closing date, and had to get some special dispensation, as it were, before my application was accepted; a late fee, or something of the sort, had to be paid. However, the exam. came round within a few weeks, and I can truthfully say that I enjoyed practically every minute of it. It was a long exam., an exam. for gentlemen; one was treated as a gentleman by the examiners, with the possible exception of one neurologist, but even that too was rather fun. My feeling at the end of it all was grave disappointment. Here was I, with an M.D. in Psychological Medicine and a D.P.M. still not knowing anything about the mind and its abnormalities, or even how to get down to providing any real help for the psychoneurotic patients. I thought to myself: 'I was nearer achieving the latter ambition working in general practice than I am here with all my "qualifications".'

I mentioned these bitter reflections to one of the junior Resident Medical Officers at Bethlem, a man who had studied some of the clinical work for the examination with me and given me a little coaching. He said: 'Shut up, don't talk to anybody like this! They will not only think you have got some dud qualifications, but they will think that we all have, that qualifications in psychiatry are dud, whereas look at the incredible amount of work we have had to swot up. Nobody would believe the amount one has to study for this, and here you are going about, giving the impression that it is all nothing or rubbish.' Well, I did not think it was nothing or rubbish. It definitely was science all right, but the point was it did not help one sufficiently to understand the real clinical problems nor to help the neurotic sufferer.

Throughout the time I had spent at Bethlem, I naturally heard much about various branches of psychology that were not pre-scribed for the examination. Besides McDougall, Kretschmer, Bleuler and other classics, mention had occasionally been made of people like Freud, Jung, Adler, Groddeck, perhaps even Wil-helm Reich. The references to Freud in particular had been as though to a very low comedian, but one who, like the low comedian, was always the soul of the party. Perhaps this man was trying to tell us something which we had left out. I had completely finished my study of the classifical authors and of the orthodox prescribed teaching, and where was I? Many of the Medical Officers took the opportunity now and again to make fun of Freud. I had used this technique very successfully at my M.D. examination. The method is as follows: having mentioned the psychopathological inter-pretation of practically every other important writer, one pauses a bit and hints that there are, of course, other views. The examiner asks for an example, you smile patronisingly and say with ever-so-slight a snigger: 'Well, of course, Freud says so-an-so.' Then everybody laughs a bit, and it makes for good feeling all round and an assurance of success. The only place where none of us has any success is when it comes to ameliorating a case of neurosis. I did not find the situation altogether gratifying, but I find it more gratifying to reflect that to-day these methods would not prove so successful. There are nowadays few psychiatrists who have so little respect for Freudian theory, though the old attitude may still linger on amongst the less enlightened.

Immediately I had finished with Bethlem, I obtained a post at the Tavistock Clinic, which was then situated in Tavistock Square. I had previously come to know Dr. Crichton-Miller, the Director, and he had asked me to join the Clinic several months before, but I told him that I would prefer to wait until I had finished with Bethlem. To this he agreed. For Dr. Crichton-Miller, the essential qualification to become a member of his staff was not psychiatric training, but general practice. This put him up enormously in my estimation; I felt he knew what he was talking about. I should here mention, for the benefit of those not acquainted with the domestic mind of the profession, that from the point of view of specialisation, to have been associated with general practice is often a stigma. This is a travesty of true valuation. It would be more appropriate to regard a knowledge of general practice as indispensable. That is why Crichton-Miller's attitude was so refreshing. When one asked him what methods he advocated or what guidance he offered, his reply was a very catholic one. He said: 'I don't care what you do, only get your patients better.' In short, it was eclecticism *par excellence*.

At the Tavistock Clinic one had ample opportunity to study psychoneurotic cases just as one pleased, in one's own time. One would arrange to see a patient two or three times a week for hourly sessions, encourage him to give details of his symptoms, take the complete case history, then go on investigating for as long as one felt there was anything to find out. It was all very interesting, and I have no doubt that some good results accrued. Everybody was doing his best. After I had been there a considerable time, I was rather surprised to find that a colleague of mine had transferred his activities to the Children's Department. This set me wondering. I met him on the stairs one day, and asked him why he had changed. He said: 'One does not get any results with these adults, they are absolutely fixed and rigid, just take up your time, and you go on for months and years and nothing happens.' 'Don't you think so, So-and-So?' he called out to another physician who was listening-in higher up the stairs. The other man confirmed his opinion. He

continued: 'With children you can get some return for your lab-
ours. They are still at a malleable stage of life. You talk to their
parents, point out what is wrong, and get the parents to treat them
differently, to understand them better. Work with children is
really worth while. I cannot say I ever did any good with adults.'
    Perhaps it was in a spirit of compromise between adults and
children, in these earliest days at the Clinic, that I elected to see,
or allowed to be foisted upon me, a recalcitrant girl of fourteen
years of age. She had refused any help from anyone, was violently
hostile, full of hate, and a hundred per cent unco-operative and
rebellious. She was brought there by an aunt only under extreme
duress. I remember her being pushed into the room where I was
sitting waiting for her, and told she would have to stay an hour. She
refused my invitation to sit down, refused to do anything she was
told, would not even look at me, and stamped off to the window, out
of which she gazed all the time. I had understood that the reason
why it was so imperative, in spite of these circumstances, that she
should have some psychotherapy, was that she was suffering from
acute gonorrhoea and refused point-blank to go to a venereal clinic,
or to any doctor, or to have any treatment whatsoever.
    I just sat in my chair and talked to her back throughout the hour.
I cannot remember what I talked about, but I knew my object
was to get some lessening of her resistance, at least to me. I probably produced all the arguments I could think of in favour of her
rebellious attitude, said how right it was that one should express
one's feelings as she was doing; all feelings particularly those of
rebellion, would not be there without cause; the world, or somebody or something, must indeed have treated her very badly, and
that was why she could not help feeling as she did, and so on and
so forth.
    At first, I got a few angry stampings from her, but gradually
she became calmer, and though she persisted in keeping her back to
me and looking out of the window, I knew sooner or later that she
had begun to listen. Two days later, more or less the same thing,
but finally, when I invited her to come and sit down, she came and
sat on the floor not far from my feet. Before long, either at that
session or the next, still with her back to me, she leant her head
against my knee. I did not stop her, as one would have done under
other circumstances. The next session, about her third or fourth,

it was amusing to see that she arrived quite differently dressed. She was in her Sunday best, spruced up with high-heeled shoes, she had even washed her face and done her hair. I smiled inwardly; I knew the thing was working.

Presently, she told me about herself. She had no mother, her father was apparently a bad character and a drunkard; it was he who had seduced her and given her the gonorrhoea. I thought, small wonder at her psychopathic reactions. Of course, I knew how to use her transference to me. I fixed up for her attendance at the venereal clinic, and she went, voluntarily, in good heart. She was going to tell me all about it next time. At the end of the following session, which in any case I had intended to be one of the last of the series, she refused to go when her hour was up, or to let me leave the room. Finally, as I tried to pass her, she put her back to the door. I talked to her for a little longer, and tried to persuade her. She moved away, and I made an attempt to leave, but at this, she suddenly flung her arms round my neck and smothered my face with passionate kisses before I could make my escape, fervently hoping that there was no infectious accompaniment to her local contagion. This was after little more than a week of seeing her, and it confirmed me in my reluctance to treat very young people. Their powers of control, their ego, are insufficiently in charge of the emotional situation for one to be able to rely upon their conforming to the rules of treatment, and I found it difficult to combine the science of therapeutic technique with more than a modicum of discipline.

Then there was that quiet little Jewess from Stepney who complained of the solitary symptom of chronic headache. The reason her doctor had the hunch that it was psychogenic and sent her to me was that its onset coincided with the date of her engagement to marry six months ago. Since then it had never left her. It was important to this girl that her ideals should remain intact in the face of all disrupting realities. She had a conventional ideal of marriage as the initiation to a love-life never previously experienced in any form or degree. The concept included all the paraphernalia of a white wedding, symbolising purity, and she even conceived of herself as carrying a bouquet of lilies—everything pure white as befitted a high-principled virgin. This she declared she certainly was, and stuck to the statement through thick and thin, despite obvious resistances to the process of free association of thought.

In due course, in *fact* it took many weeks, it transpired that it was the superhuman strain of maintaining this belief that was responsible for the perpetual headache. The difficulties involved in repression became more understandable when it came to light that in the neighbourhood of her home, she almost daily passed some young man with whom she had experienced at least some degree of sexual intimacy, and even occasionally a pretty full degree. Over and above this, the following story finally emerged: she and her fiancé were in the habit of meeting at least three times a week in her parents' flat on the upper floor of a tenement building. On each of these occasions he would depart late and she would accompany him down the stairs to a dark passage, where they were in the habit of having complete intercourse in the form of *coitus interruptus*. The thought may occur to one that the emotional strain of *coitus interruptus* might well account for the chronic headache, but the truth was that this had been practised for several months *before* the engagement, and had never led to any such symptom as headache until the day she became engaged and the engagement was made public. The coincidence in time between this and the headache strongly suggested that it was due to (at least as a precipitating factor) the psychological mechanism of conflict leading to repression. This theory was practically confirmed by the fact that when all these confessions had emerged and she could no longer maintain the repression, when she had readjusted her mind, and needed no longer to deny to herself the truth, the headaches vanished completely. Simple cases like this were the exception rather than the rule, but therapeutic success, however exceptional, compensated for a lot of relatively unrewarding work.

One had the common spectacle of seeing colleagues who were keen and who worked hard at the Clinic, eventually drop out, often quite suddenly; they would take up some other work, go back to general practice, or enter the asylum service. It gave one the impression that they had tried to understand and to cure neurosis, and had, despite their painstaking efforts, finally given it up as a bad job. All this might have been very disturbing. I knew that psychology was the key to the riddle of much more than a special branch of medicine. For me, it was going to be everything, it was going to take the place of every other scientific interest. That *I* should give it up was absolutely out of the question; it was going to be much more to me than trying to help people as best one could at the Tavistock Clinic. Admittedly, a lot of the patients tended to become extremely chronic; they attended two or three times a week, month in and month out, even year in and year out. Admittedly, one was quite used to this sort of thing in general practice. Every general practitioner faces with equanimity the prospect of patients coming weekly or twice weekly for decades, or for the rest of their lives, but this was not the idea at the Tavistock Clinic. Suddenly a new woman physician arrived who improved statistical records enormously. She saw a succession of patients, some of them chronics, who very soon ceased to attend. They were put down as cured. I more than suspected that what they were cured of was seeing the doctor, nothing else.

This state of affairs was not satisfactory, and I had at the back of my mind known all along what I was going to do about it, what my next move would be. I sought an interview with the then President of the British Psycho-Analytical Society, and discussed with him my programme of undergoing a complete psycho-analytical training. After all, what had I sold three-quarters of my general practice and half my income for? I was prepared to apply myself with unremitting diligence in the pursuit of my research. I was told that the first item on the programme was that I should subject myself to a training analysis. I had been forewarned of this, and it was the aspect of the course that appealed to me least. I said to him: 'What about the rest of the course? Don't we go to lectures, don't you prescribe suitable reading? What books should I get?' and so on. He said to my astonishment: 'Don't read anything. We recommend no reading. When you are analysed, you will find that you read the book of your own unconscious, and, to begin with at least, that is the only book advisable.' The expense involved in paying for one's own analysis was a serious consideration. I said I thought I could afford to go perhaps twice or three times a week. He simply shook his head. He said to me: 'When you hear of people attending for analysis two or three times a week, you will know that it is not psychoanalysis. Your attendance must be five consecutive days at least.'

All this was not so devastating as might have been supposed. On the contrary, I found it rather exhilarating. Perhaps here was something at last which would supply the key to the scriptures. However, I almost fell foul of him before the end of the interview, partly because I had, very characteristically, kept something under my hat. He began to go through a list of analysts, male and female, who had vacancies and would be prepared to take me on. He also mentioned their fees. I listened until he said the name of Professor J. C. Flugel. Only then did I interrupt him and say: 'Actually I decided I would go to Flugel ever since I attended his lectures at University College a year ago.' The doctor put down his pen and said to me: 'Why didn't you say so before?' My answer was a perfectly simple one, but did not mitigate his annoyance: 'Well, first I wanted to see whether or not *you* would mention him.' After all, choosing an analyst is a most important matter; the analysis may continue for a year or more, may make a difference to one's entire life, and everything connected with it. I did not at that time know that it was not a question of 'may make a difference', that it was certain to make a difference, and I had no conception of how great the difference would be. How could I have?

A second time I annoyed the President before I left: I thought I might gain some kudos by telling him that I was already treating patients at the Tavistock Clinic. Again he put down his pen, looked seriously at me, and said: 'Have you not considered the stigma of being associated with such a place?' Strangely enough, I was more delighted than crestfallen at this remark, which seemed to show me something of the bias which one expected to find between the members of one rival institution and another, but which I hardly anticipated in the President of the British Psycho-Analytical Society. I was delighted that he was so human. He was not favourably impressed by my obvious happiness, which he mistook for levity. Actually I was tactless and foolish enough to display lightheartedness throughout the interview. It was due to my exhilaration and excitement at what I was feeling to be the real initiation of my true and final specialisation. It was disapointing to realise that the leading psychoanalyst and specialist in interpretation could so confidently misinterpret it. He said as much. That was *too* human. Anyhow, I rushed straight off to the Tavistock Clinic, and hilariously repeated to a room full of assembled colleagues the President's remark about 'the stigma of being associated with such a place.' How extroverted I was becoming—or pretendnig to be!

Several of them returned the compliment, and asked if I had ever considered the stigma of being associated with the British Psycho-Analytical Society. Well, stigma or not, such an association at that stage of my studies and investigations seemed to me absolutely inevitable. I could not have been satisfied with life or with the turn my life had taken towards this interest in psychological work, and at the same time have neglected to investigate and to experience everything that psychoanalysis had to offer. Fate was treading me into her pattern.

While I launched myself into a personal analysis, I nevertheless still continued my work at the Tavistock Clinic which, in the light of what I was beginning to learn through my analytical attendances, began to take on a fresh interest for me. I may have tried to imitate the methods of my analyst when exercising the new technique upon my Tavistock patients. Crichton-Miller had said: 'I don't care what you do, only try to make them better.' I now felt that I was learning something of a new technique for trying to make them better. I could, at the same time, see what it yielded in me and what it yielded in them.

At a meeting of psychologists and psychoanalysts before I had really launched upon my own analysis, I was telling a man of the programme the President had prescribed for me, and raising objections to it. I mentioned that I was not aware of any psychoses, neuroses or complexes in myself (forgetting at the time that I was subject to neuralgic attacks). It turned out that this man had himself been analysed, and my remarks caused him amusement and laughter. He said very meaningfully: 'Don't worry, you soon will be!' I said: 'I soon will be?' He replied: 'You will soon be aware of the whole lot, all the complexes; every neurosis and every psychosis. You wait!' and he laughed again. I was delighted. This was just what I wanted. Of course! How *could* anyone truly understand these odd things unless he discovered them right inside himself.

One of the first things that amazed me in the early weeks of my own analysis was the sudden and totally unexpected revelation of the meaning of a particular dream symbol, a revelation which would never have occurred to me without the analyst's help, and yet, when he said it, it was as clear and convincing as any discovery one makes oneself and sees before one's own eyes. The dream had nightmare qualities: I was with a tennis player whom I had never been able to beat, and who had partnered me at tournaments away from London. He was a man who reminded me, by dint of one or two characteristics only, of my deceased father, though I had never been conscious of this till I associated to his appearance in the dream. We were on holiday or something together, we had adjoining bedrooms, it was night, and I had just gone to bed. I got the nightmare feeling that something peculiar was going to happen; and sure enough, the outside bedroom door, the one into the passage, opened stealthily, and through a crack there came into the room a pecular little figure, like a gnome or pixie. Suddenly it darted towards me. I was terrified and screamed, with the familiar choked feeling, to my friend for help. Before he could come to my rescue, the figure, now rather Puck-like, grinning and breathing my name, had leapt on the rail at the foot of my bed. As I cowered under the sheets, it sprinkled me with some powder or fluid from what might have been a salt cellar. I caught a glimpse of the alarmed face of my friend, and awoke in terror.

To me, at that time, this little nightmare was entirely incomprehensible. It was still incomprehensible when I told it, laughing, to my analyst at the session. After I had produced the associations of thought that this particular friend reminded me of my father, and had dwelt upon the dream as best I could, still without a clue as to the nature of the little, grotesque, terrifying apparition, the analyst said quietly: 'It is a penis.' Instantly, of course, I knew the whole thing. It was none the less amazing to me. Had I been told such a dream and been asked who in this whole world would be least likely ever to dream such a thing, I believe I would have said that that person was me. It seemed to me as foreign to my psychology as anything could possibly be—which only goes to show that there are stranger things in our unconscious than are dreamed of in our conscious estimate of ourselves.

This was a classical nightmare, a dream in which the repressed feminine component creates its wish-fulfilling phantasy of sexual attention from the father, attention to the repressed, unconscious and repudiated desires; at that unconscious level it has all the advantages of feminine gratification together with incestuous gratification, which of course means that it belongs to the Oedipus level of emotional development. Now, this phantasy of inverted

Oedipus gratification is utterly repressed and utterly foreign to the conscious levels of the psyche, in fact the ego levels of the psyche, unconscious as well as conscious, are more than repudiating it. They would regard its triumph as their annihilation. That is why, when in the dream feminine desire for gratification is gaining ground, they, the ego levels, are anticipating being annihilated. They are the levels with which the dreamer identifies himself, the other is the level of incestuous, inverted gratification which the dreamer has repressed, repudiated and disowned. He has no conception that such a world has anything whatsover to do with him. It would be his most firmly rejected enemy; and here it has come as a phantasy during his sleep. Therefore it is felt as some intrusion from outside, an intrusion that is going to do incalculable harm, an intrusion that is terrifying, annihilating. And the terror of the nightmare is that he feels that he is powerless to stop it; it is gaining the upper hand; all he can do is the most desperate thing a sleeper can do, and that is to awake.

With the analyst's mention of the word 'penis', all this was revealed to me. I discovered in a flash the incredible truth which I could no longer deny: that there were elements in me which no amount of reading or persuasion or study of others or anything else in the world would ever have persuaded me could possibly exist there at all; and here, with this dream interpretation, I did not need any persuasion, it was obvious. All the motions of the dream in this new light were completely consistent, understandable, and inevitable. I had received my first introduction to an entirely new world, a world which no amount of persuasion would ever have made me believe could possibly exist anywhere . . . and here I had seen it . . . and lo, it was in me all the time! Incidentally even one little dream like this, when fully understood gives the dreamer a better understanding both of homosexuality *and* of the normal horror of homosexuality, than any amount of reading and theory can ever give him!

It was only at a later stage of my analysis that I discovered that one of the determinants in the dream-friend was none other than my analyst. All three persons, the tennis player, my father and this analyst, were bald-headed. Thus the particular dream figure had been chosen on this account to represent both my father and my analyst. So the transference of father-affect to analyst was already under way, but was too heavily censored for me to see it at that stage of my analysis.

Naturally, this was not the only change in my orientation that the early weeks of analysis produced. This was a sample of legitimate internal change, the sort of change that makes for insight and genuine analytical progress. Analysis should ideally be confined to such changes, at least until it has run its course. One of the dangers, one which I think is commonly over-estimated, is that an analysand does not always obey the rules and confine his analytical movement to an internal one. We have got into the habit throughout life, in fact life may be said to be identical *with* the habit, of discharging our unrepressed or released energy, our libido and our aggression, in mobile relationships to environment. In other words, our drives and instinct gratifications habitually express themselves in extroverted activities, not normally confining themselves to introverted or intrapsychic activities. *The behaviour of life might be defined as activity, very often symptomatic activity, instigated by tensions within the psyche and designed to reduce or relieve those tensions.* Every advance of science helps to confirm that life, our behaviour, is nothing more than this. There is no gainsaying the compulsion of the forces within any more than that of the forces without, such as the movement of the sun and the Earth. Hence the title of this book, *being lived. . . .* Thus, it is not surprising if the tendency in analysis is for the analysand to use up libidinal energy, released from repression, by discharging it in some form of extra-analytical activity.

CHAPTER XIII

LOVE AND MARRIAGE

IN in the earliest weeks of my analysis, I began to realise what a frustration the close association with my mother (I was still living with her) had become, and I regret to say that I became less successful in repressing and suppressing the feelings of irritation with which I had long reacted to her motherly care and limited possessiveness. Although I had an average number of friends, including a little retinue of girl friends, it had never previously struck me that nobody had mattered or could possibly matter like my mother mattered. One of the very early fruits of analysis was that I began to feel this need not always be the case, and I became unwittingly a little more open about my feeling of frustration than I had previously been.

At that time, my mother had ceased to keep house for Dr. Saunderson and myself in the practice at North London. She and I had left the premises to him and his housekeeper, and had instead taken a little flat not far from the Tavistock Clinic where I was in the habit of spending my afternoons. This was the domestic situation under which I was working and being analysed.

The internal movements that were taking place as a result of analysis were, I think, subconsciously beginning to make me feel that drastic changes would come about, not only in my internal mental life, but also in my actual life, in my environment. I had not faced up to any sort of clear appreciation of what they might be, but I sensed somehow that they would probably be something that had not been dreamed of in my philosophy.

I was still in the very early stages of my introduction to this new, amazing and unsuspected world that lay within myself, when one afternoon I returned home from the Tavistock Clinic, and found present a most unusual visitor. I was accustomed to finding friends of my mother in to tea, I was even accustomed to meeting an occasional young lady under these circumstances, daughters or nieces of Anglo-Indian relatives, friends and acquaintances, but this visitor took my breath away on the instant. It was a girl of about twenty-two years, seated on a pouffe near the foot of my mother's chair. They were having tea. I first saw a mop of light golden hair, and then, as she jerked her head round attractively, a fresh pink and white complexion, blue eyes, and a very genial, happy, smiling face. There was a 'presence' that held me spellbound. There was something more than poetry about her contours and her movements. There was a quality which might be summed up in the term 'life', young life, ripe life, life that was synonymous with sex and reproduction. It is impossible to describe these attributes in a person, the whole thing is so predominantly subjective. The old song has it very well when it says, 'I took one look at you, that's all I meant to do; and then, my heart stood still.' The lyricist does not go into psychoanalytical detail to explain why the heart stood still, but most of us can more or less understand it emotionally, if not intellectually. I came into this room as I had done hundreds of times before, and this was the only occasion on which my breathing had been arrested and my heart stood still. What was it? Was it the charming, happy young lady, or was it the fruits of that stage of my analysis and the fact that the analyst had just left for his summer vacation? Perhaps it was a bit of both.

I believe the truth is that I was married at that instant, in a fraction of a second. Far away was it for me to think of such a matter in terms of 'marriage'. Good gracious, in those days I held the scientific view that the whole institution of matrimony should be abolished. It was an unwarranted, religion-induced interference with the natural laws of sexual attraction and the natural laws of psychological and physiological, especially physiological, reaction of one person to another. We were creatures of these laws and should follow them (so I held), and not muck them about by introducing unwarranted, irrelevant principles, religious or otherwise. Nature should be good enough for us, and our realities should fit it; anything else was nonsense. So my 'marriage' to this unexpected visitor was just simply instant marriage. Of course, there was no necessity to have the bridal night immediately! I could wait any length of time. My powers of bearing frustration had been said, even by my analyst, to be phenomenal. Perhaps I could bear it better because I knew quite confidently that a bridal night was inevitable; the apparition of this girl had told me so . . . and with whom. It did not seem to me to matter much how things began; but why waste unnecessary time? Therefore, when she assisted in carrying the tea things from the lounge to the kitchen and we met there away from my mother's eye, I simply said: 'When can you come dancing with me?' She replied briefly: 'On Thursday night. That is my evening off; I will get a late pass.' (She was a probationer nurse at University College Hospital). I said: 'I will call for you at eight o'clock. We will go to a night club.' She did not express a lot of enthusiasm, but showed her willingness and looked slightly bemused.

We had an extraordinarily hilarious evening at the night club. Here was an occasion and here was company in which I could let myself go completely. We drank a magnum of champagne between us and danced everything, with her laughing and singing most of the time. Everything was completely on the positive side so far as my reactions to her were concerned, no criticisms or doubts whatsoever assailed me. This is a very happy state of affairs psychologically. I mention it because I am sure that I must have had part-reactions of this same nature towards a succession of girls, but I could not think of any instance where there had been no qualification to them, where my ego had said: 'There is no hesitating or bargaining with this. Your instincts can just go straight ahead. Consequences, if any, are beside the point; in any case, it is inevitable, inevitable all the way.'

What did I want with an analyst any more? Let him stay away on his blessed summer holiday, three months in Scandinavia or wherever else he chose, and write his books. I would be happy enough with this delightful, exhilarating girl. Practically every bit of her off-time was spent in my company. She dropped all other tentative attachments and I dropped all mine. We had been living thus in a state of exceptional, if not unique, happiness for several weeks or months when she suddenly indicated to me that perhaps marriage would not be a bad idea. I was a little surprised; I had made it clear to her, as always to every one of my friends, that I did not see any sense in the introduction of artificiality into personal relationships. Here, between Celia and me, was a per-fectly natural situation, which would of course develop naturally if left to nature. Even if it were a question of having children, I think I was prepared to ignore the conventions. I would have felt more in character, with family and all, however large, if it could have been regarded as a natural phenomenon to which con-

ventional ideas of marriage and so on were entirely irrelevant.
Marriage, I held, was necessary for unethical people, wolves and
cads and so on from whom women needed to be protected, but for a
person like myself, to whom it would be anathema to treat any
person, particularly a girl, shabbily, this binding-in-wedlock-
business was not only superfluous, but out of character and almost
insulting. Nature should be allowed to take its course and we,
the man as well as the woman, sharing the same boat, should
accept the consequences. And here was this lovely girl, with
nothing to fear as far as I was concerned, more or less suggesting
that it might be just as well to get married. Perhaps this was my
first slight disappointment in her, but there was no hesitation
in my reaction. My stand was that with a woman whom I love and
who loves me, her true wishes are my law. 'Of course, my darling,
if you want us to marry, we will marry, or anything else you like.
You know I belong to you, marriage or no marriage, but if you
prefer the conventional seal of marriage, you must have whatever makes you happy.'

My analyst had returned from his holiday, and I took the young
lady round to see him. He seemed to me somewhat nonplussed
when I phoned him up and told him about it. Indeed, he gave me
the impression that he was quite flabbergasted, all of a dither; he
hemmed and ha-ed, but presently saw my determination, and con-
sented to see us. I called there with her in my car. He came out
and I introduced them. I stood back on the pavement outside his
house, and watched with amusement how he was entirely cap-
tivated. He was all over her and quite forgot my presence. It seemed
to me that I would almost have to drag him away. I think she
guessed that he was rather an important person to get on the right
side of, more important than was apparent. This contact convinced
him, like nothing else would have done, that her union and mine was
inevitable, that it was no good making any attempt to defer it until analysis was over. One has only to picture this lovely radiant,
yet, self-possessed girl as she was in those days to realise with half
an eye, if one is a heterosexual male, that union, mating, immediate mating, was indeed inevitable.

Later on, however, when I interviewed the President of the
Society, he blew up instantly. He almost shouted at me: 'You
fool! Have you no insight? Don't you see what you have done?

You have left the man (analyst) for the woman!' Then, later, he soliloquised: 'I suppose it will all have to simmer down before you will be fit to get on with your analysis.' I could see that I had received my first really bad mark in my relationship to the Psycho-Analytical Society. I could see that in this man's view, analysis was the one and only thing that mattered. Marriages, families, children, everything in the ordinary reality world was of no account or consequence in comparison with the one and only worth-while purpose of one's life, and that was to achieve a complete and successful analysis. I wondered if he was right. However, it gave me food for thought.

I have often subsequently throughout my post-analytical career subjected people, especially patients, to the following little homily in answer to questions as to whether this or that would do them good or be a good adjustment in their lives. I have said: 'When a sailor puts his arm round a girl in the park, he is probably by this "symptomatic act" doing himself some good. He is, in part at least, gratifying his impulse or preparing to do so, preparing to relieve his otherwise uncomfortable psychological state of tension. In short, his behaviour may be very therapeutic; *but*, and this is the point, however therapeutic, it is not analysis. I have no doubt that all behaviour of all people throughout their lives is, generally speaking, designed to relieve their tensions, fundamentally their instinct tensions, and thereby to make them feel more comfortable, happier and healthier, but we are talking of behaviour, the activities of people. None of this is analysis; it is just life. Maybe it is therapeutically better than analysis, maybe the sailor's behaviour in the park is more immediately beneficial than analysis would be. In so far as we behave naturally, we may not require analysis for our immediate health and comfort, perhaps we have found a better way; but generally speaking, the reason people come to analysis, the reason analysis was ever instituted at all, is that these people have not found a good enough, a perfect enough, way of curing themselves, or relieving their tensions by their behaviour and their adjustment to environment. It is failure to achieve this by the simple and natural expedient of behaviour that makes insight, understanding, in short analysis, desirable or necessary. Eventually, in the light of the insight and the understanding, some other attempt may be found to be desirable or necessary.'

I would extend this theory, as I have done in a recent paper, and say this: So long as instinctual behaviour is achieving gratification, the psychological and physiological processes of life go on healthily and happily and the faculty of thought and intelligence is not called for at all. If this had been the condition throughout the process of evolution, living organisms would, at the most, be limited to instinctual or reflex activity, and the brain (meaning by that the intelligence) would never have been so much as initiated, it would not have been born, in short, there would have been no such thing as psychology, and perhaps no such thing as evolution beyond a certain point. If a dog or any animal in nature has all its instincts gratified and encounters no frustrations, well it just has its instincts gratified and that becomes the be-all and end-all of its life. Maybe if, whenever an organism felt hunger, food was immediately put into its mouth, it would, far from developing or evolving, even regress back to a stage when it did not possess any muscles except those necessary for swallowing food. Even a caterpillar is a higher product of evolution than that.

My thesis is that it is the failure to gratify an instinct, the failure to achieve adequate 'therapeutic' relief of tension by one's behaviour, the presence of something that frustrates this, which alone leads the organism to call upon other less immediately gratifying faculties which it may or may not have in reserve. If it has not got them in reserve, this situation of frustration creates a necessity for them, and, I am convinced, initiates their creation, really their development, from whatever energies and faculties within the organism are already present. The stages of events are, therefore, first that instinct gratification is frustrated, second that a stage of consequent discomfort or tension is unrelieved and tends to increase. This is the stage of 'illness' that calls for, or mobilises, all the faculties within the organism in an endeavour to overcome the frustration. It is really a battle of life and death, for if instincts are not gratified, the organism will get more and more ill and perish. Thus, the so-called higher faculties of the mind, the intelligence, the ability to think, are born out of a state of frustration, discomfort or potential illness. Their further development or even their utilisation, depends upon a recurrence of frustrations, that is to say of situations which fail to gratify instincts and to relieve tensions.

In so far as we can achieve full satisfaction, relief of tension, happiness, by our behaviour, we may be regarded as making successful adjustments in our environment, and we will only use those faculties which are necessary to ensure this gratification, health and happiness. Other faculties, such as those of intelligence, particularly psychological insight, will only come into being in so far as they have to, that is to say, in so far as we are failing to manage adequately without them.

Thus, there were grounds for distress on the part of the President of the psychoanalysts on my behalf, for in so far as I was succeeding in achieving satisfactory internal and external adjustment and happiness in my relationship to my new-found love, in so far as this was destined to fill my life and make me healthy and happy, in so far would I find analysis superfluous. I would not be asking for it, any more than the sailor in the park would be asking for it. It is health, comfort, happiness and gratification that the organism is after, not the development of intelligence, analytical or otherwise. The President might have said to me: 'Perhaps you will be so happy this way, in your new marriage, that you will naturally spend all your time and money on that and be glad to do so, and wonder why on earth such a thing as analysis, or for that matter any intellectual interest whatsoever, was ever invented.'

Well, if this were true, what on earth had I been doing all the rest of my life up to that moment? In the course of analysis it had become more and more plain to me what I had been doing or not doing. I had been frustrated by my attachment to my mother and had unwittingly been trying to cope with that frustration, blindly and inappropriately.

Now, the problem was would my new-found love so gratify all my needs in life that I would have no further use for my research, nor indeed for my intelligence, except in so far as it were necessary to earn enough money to maintain the material basis for this wonderful love relationship.

And, if the answer to this were in the affirmative, if my happiness would be complete by virtue of my new love adjustment, was there indeed any need for regret? If the aim of one's life's endeavours, behaviouristic and psychological, is to achieve as great a happiness as possible, I, having achieved it, should be congratulated all round, as well as congratulating myself, not

stigmatised by the President of the Psycho-Analytical Society as a
fool who had made a ghastly mistake, Well, of course, the President
was a peculiar chap; he had made a religion, a god, of psycho-
analytical research, a very poor substitute, I thought at that time,
for the happiness to be found in living a robust, passionate,
emotional life. It seemed that his criterion was: analysis is the one
good, anything and everything that interferes with it is therefore
bad . . . and perhaps happiness worst of all! What an extraordinary
position to get to. Well, to hell with the lot of them! In any case,
here was I inexorably caught up in the big, emotional drive of life;
the tide of nature had swept me along this way; it was destiny,
call it what you like, there was no alternative for me, at least not
at present.

I turned my back on them all, the President, Glover, Flugel,
and all the psychoanalysts. Could I convince myself that I had
found something better? In a sense at that time I needed no aid to
conviction. Celia and I were in each other's arms, and that was all
there was to it. She wanted the marriage; the marriage must go
ahead. Why should it prove such a disaster, as the President's
rude words had implied? After all, even analysts get married.
Indeed, I had researched so long, perhaps in the wrong direction;
maybe, after all, this was the answer right under my nose, the
answer which had been too close for me to see all these years of
my life with my ridiculous eyes focused upon the horizon. What an
idiot I was! Here was nature all around me, not only exemplified
in the human species, but in every living organism, animal and
vegetable, everyone of them telling me this answer from the day
I was born, and I had been neglecting it all, looking at distant
horizons, the riddle of the universe! Indeed, I must be the maddest
fool that ever was, or at least the blindest. I and my research!
and, of all things, into the nature of the mind! That made it even
more laughable. It had taken a young girl, a natural product of
healthy nature, who had hardly ever bothered with science or even
with thought, to tell me the answer quite simply: 'Marriage'!

Well, get married I did.

I must say this for the genuineness of my researches before it
is too late to say it. Throughout all these studies of mine, both
while in general practice and subsequently at Bethlem Royal
Hospital, and throughout all the time I spent at the Tavistock

Clinic, it had never once crossed my mind, not even when I obtained an M.D. and D.P.M., that this psychological research, leading as it did to specialisation in psychiatry, had or would ever have any connection whatsoever with income, with earning money. My ideal was to know and understand the mind, not to prostitute my precious enthusiasm for research to economic needs.

So it was that towards the end of my first year's work at the Tavistock, when I had been appointed a physician on their staff, it came to me as a surprise when a senior colleague, walking along the street beside me, suddenly said: 'Well, Berg, when are you going to take a room in Harley Street?' I can still remember the shock I got at his suggestion. I looked at him and just muttered: 'Harley Street?' and thought to myself 'What on earth had Harley Street to do with me?' He dilated on the subject, and pointed out how one could get an address in Harley Street for a mere forty pounds a year, provided of course one never actually practised there. It was a good beginning to have an address; it got one's name coupled with the auspicious address in the directory and in the telephone book, and eventually, when a patient turned up, the landlord would accommodate one, as long as it did not happen very often. If it *did* happen very often, one would go one better and get the part-time use of a room, even if it were only for once a week; naturally, that was a much more expensive proposition.

Now that I was about to get married, a different attitude towards my professional position was bound to intrude and claim attention; the question of economics. I did not want it to intrude. Since I had left Enfield, and more especially since I had made psychological and psychiatric studies my main interest, recreation and hobby, I had not found it difficult to ignore the economic side of my activities. Why could not things just go on like this? Celia and I could be together, live together, keep house together where and when it suited our financial ability or the money in my pocket, just in the same way as we could dine at a cheap café or have a beano at a night club according to how well off I felt at the time, according to adjustment of inclination and financial ability. This seemed to me a natural way of going on. If we lived together, that too would be natural; where and how we lived would, of course, have to be according to our purse. If we chose to have children, then we would naturally have to meet the necessary expenses. I did not see the point of making any formal and artificial changes. Everything, I felt, should be just natural reaction and natural adjustment, including economics; but I was not surprised that the lady's viewpoint was a little different, rather more conventional. After all, the narrow way these girls had been educated, what more could one expect!

It was not entirely pleasing, nor entirely displeasing, that she showed a tendency to make what I felt was an unnecessary hoo-ha about everything. Engagement ring—all right, that was a bit of fun; a great, formal wedding with everybody dressed up and an enormous choral service—well, perhaps that too was tolerably good fun. When my analyst, knowing my views about such ceremonies, inadvertently expressed a little surprise, I replied cryptically: 'Well, the whole idea and institution of matrimony is such crazy nonsense that one might as well make it obviously nonsensical by beating tom-toms, singing psalms or making any other sort of irrelevant noises, rituals and rubbish. I quite approve of this rubbish, because it might otherwise seem as though one were pretending that marriage is sense. The nonsense that is marriage might as well be made obvious and conspicuous, and one might as well enjoy it, like a fancy-dress party.'

A difficulty which I immediately encountered was linked up with my lack of insight into what, to me, were unobvious emotional relationships to other women. The other woman, in this instance, was my mother. To my amazement, as soon as she heard of the engagement, she almost had a nervous breakdown. I was most perplexed and disappointed. In the days of Sylvia, it had seemed to me that my mother was not only quite amenable to my marriage (with Sylvia) but even seemed to be advocating it. I can see now that the fact was that this young woman, Sylvia, was far more emotionally attached to my mother, especially while she was living in the North London house with us, than she was to me. Perhaps in a sense it was my mother to whom she was married, and I do not think she would have had much use for me, at least not much passionate use. Mother could have tolerated my marriage to her very well. Was it the tendency of mothers to want their sons to have marriages that were not marriages at all in the true passionate and sexual sense? What fond mothers really want is to be able to give their son some part of themselves, some woman, perhaps a homosexual woman, a mother-fixated young woman who needs mother in the shape of themselves most of all and who will, as it were, accept the son as part of the bargain. Well, I suppose it is all very natural from the point of view of the psychology of a widowed and ageing lady. Perhaps there is no way of making the various needs of various people, linked to each other on some old and should-be-outworn emotional basis, dovetail into one another.

Here was my poor, devoted mother who had slaved for me from the time of my birth, almost wrecked mentally and physically at the prospect of my marrying this scintillating and capable girl. Whatever could one do about it? The little bit of analysis I had had, had shown me pretty clearly, if it had shown me nothing else, that I was more married to my mother than I had ever suspected, and that such a marriage involved a frustration of one's natural sexual expression in life. Love, adult love, is physiologically designed by nature to include certain forms of behaviour and certain physiological reactions. These cannot take place if the love-object is a parent, in every way consciously and unconsciously sexually taboo, unthinkable, unwanted. Deep in the mind, whether we recognise it or not, an antagonism, a dicotomy existed between the mental attachment (in this case to my mother) and the emotional sexual drive which nature had meant to join forces with the mental for a complete, conflict-free relationship with another person. The other person should be a mate, not a mother. I had recently recognised all this more clearly than ever before, and perhaps felt an unjustified resentment against what I had hitherto accepted so gratuitously—the devotion of my mother. Recently, I heard a mother express the fond hope that her son would never leave her. I said to her: 'Sons grow up, you know! It is usually better that way. Perhaps you should have another son . . . and another.'

Of course, outwardly I pooh-poohed all my mother's objections, insisted that everything would be all right, that she would see I should be happy, and I would therefore be in a better position to make her happy. No stuff of this sort touched my mother in the slightest; it seemed as though she knew. Unfortunately, her grave reaction, amounting almost to an illness, had not passed unobserved by my fiancée. This introduced, as it were, something nasty to her mind; a little nastiness had crept in to this hitherto lovely situation, a little nastiness and a very big difficulty. Somehow or other, mother had to be banished; maybe in practice this was a possibility. One would have to find a cottage or something for her somewhere; but an unhappy mother, after our life-long happiness together, outward happiness at least, was something quite inconsistent with a happy me. How could I ever be happy with Celia or with anybody else if my poor, devoted mother, to whom I owed everything throughout my life, was unhappy and in exile? What was I letting myself in for by being disloyal to my 'scientific' ideals? The mass of objections to my situation was piling up.

The biggest difficulty, as no doubt millions of people have found before me, proved in due course to be the economic one. No sooner had the marriage been arranged, than the question arose of a place to live in together, the furnishing and establishing of it, all the expenditure and paraphernalia that were necessary to make an appropriate setting for a grand and glorious marriage. To me, it was absolutely awful—anathema. I would have lived anywhere, in a room, in a hovel, but in accordance with the available money and the prospect of money remaining available. It would have been natural for me to cut my suit according to my cloth. It soon became clear that these were not Celia's ideas. To her any such ideas would have been nonsensical, just as nonsensical as hers were to me. But after all, these were little matters, I fondly hoped, that did not necessarily affect the main issue, namely our great and all-pervading passionate love for each other. A necessary part of that love relationship, a natural part of it for me, was that all her wishes should be granted, and I should accept the consequences. There must be something to be said for her attitude, perhaps as much as there was for mine, perhaps more, for her attitude was certainly more in keeping with that of the majority of people. So off we went to Mill Hill, where I had thought of purchasing one of the small houses advertised in those days at seven hundred and fifty pounds. Not that I had seven hundred and fifty pounds; I think I possessed altogether something in the region of five hundred pounds savings, but of course one would get it on mortgage.

At Mill Hill the speculative builder to whom I was taken pooh-poohed the idea of my getting one of those small houses. He said: 'Why, those are only built for workmen; a man like you, in your position, could hardly live in a house like that; you would probably have working men each side of you.' I looked at my luscious and beautifully dressed, prospective bride. She said nothing, but I knew what she was thinking. The seven hundred and fifty pound house was out of the question. He showed me a beautiful little double-fronted, detached villa with garage, a small garden, and a large oak tree growing at the bottom of it. This property, he told me, freehold, was only one thousand, nine hundred and fifty. Oh yes, I could easily purchase it; the building society would not give more than one thousand five hundred, but he himself would grant me a second mortgage of two hundred pounds, so that I would only have to put down two hundred and fifty. The rest would all be paid in subsequent quarterly instalments. I wondered how far one could stretch eight hundred pounds per annum, but could see nothing else for it. Anyhow, it was argued, the house was suitable and in a nice position for putting up a plate if subsequently I found the need to augment my income by opening a local general practice.

The least I can say about all these arrangements is that my heart was not in it. I could feel, as it were, the chains and cords of a conventional world being tied around me. The builder rightly remarked that I could take twenty years in which to pay off the main building society mortgage. I thought to myself: 'Chains and cords for twenty years!'

It can readily be appreciated that as the economic situation grew worse, so my attention and activities had to be diverted more and more to the struggle to reach and maintain solvency. Thus, the interest and pleasure in the new-found love relationship with my wife suffered in consequence. One cannot lie happily in the arms of a girl, however lovely, while insecurity and anxiety are knocking at the door. First things first; realities have to be dealt with before we can enjoy love's sweet dream. There is no adequate gratification possible, at least not for the sane, at the expense of reality demands. This should remind us that if an infant feels insecurity in its parents' love, which is the infantile equivalent of the adult's reality situation, it will experience anxiety reactions instead of pleasure and gratification reactions, and it will inevitably grow into a neurotic.

As my reality stresses and their attendant anxieties increased, so naturally my capacity for finding happiness with my wife, with the person and the situation so closely associated with the anxiety and, as I sometimes felt, so directly responsible for it, decreased until there was a conflict between these two worlds. Love and marriage had not suceeded in providing me with the happiness-solution that had promised to 'solve all my problems', the quest for satisfaction and happiness, and so render the process of personal analysis superfluous.

Though I had begun my analysis in consequence, so far as I knew, of a drive, almost amounting to a compulsion, to understand the source and nature of other people's neuroses and sufferings, maybe always to some extent an unconscious projection of one's own, and though I had thought at one time, in the ecstasy of my new-found love, that this was a matter of more urgency and importance even than research, now, at last, I was beginning to feel the most urgent matter was the solution of my own problems, that I myself was the harassed, worried, anxiety-ridden person, and that my own case claimed priority of attention and therapy. I had been told, before analysis, that I would find the elements of every psychosis and neurosis within my own psyche, but I had not anticipated that I would find them so vividly, and experience them as a reality in my own life.

I have said previously that if a living creature has achieved, in its relationship to reality, full instinct gratification and perfect happiness, it has no need to mobilise its mental or intellectual resources. Intelligence, in fact the ego itself, is, I am sure, born of discomfort, frustration, the failure to gratify instincts, the failure to reach happiness. Then, and then only, does the necessity arise to mobilise one's resources for the purpose of overcoming frustrations, in order to relieve tension and come to rest, to comfort, gratification and happiness.

I had thought, in the full flush of my new-found love, that this was the answer that I had unconsciously been seeking, the answer that had all the time been under my very nose. I had thought, but only for a time, that happiness, however achieved, might prove to be as valuable as the struggles, strains and stresses of intellectual endeavour and research. I had evidently, though only for a time, been inclined to abandon my gods. I wondered if the pickle I was in might be regarded as the fruits of my disloyalty to them and myself. After all, I had capitulated in this marriage idea, in spite of my philosophy; love had got me first, and one thing had led to another.

During this period I attended an annual dinner at St. Thomas's Hospital. The man sitting opposite me happened to be the late Dr. John Rickman. Temporarily I recaptured something of my debonair, light-hearted mood. I made a little fun of him and his psychoanalysis. I said to him: 'I tried a bit of it, and it made a wonderful mess of my life.' He looked up at me a little quizically, and said: 'Analysis would not do much good otherwise.' and added, 'you cannot make an omelette without breaking eggs.' I have come to understand very thoroughly what he meant.

My mind became preoccupied principally with two matters almost to the exclusion of the enjoyment which I could still capture on occasions with my delightfully gay and happy young wife. The two matters were, firstly and principally, how to earn enough money to keep our heads financially above water, and secondly how to get some mental relief from the problem which my situation as a whole created for me. I could not bear the thought of acquiescing to a permanent deflection of my interest into economics and away from scientific research. Gradually, the thought began to take shape in my mind that of course the answer to all this was to resume my personal analysis. A factor in the protracted deferment of my analysis had been that it would, of course, worsen the financial situation. Analysis had to be paid for monthly. Was it not absurd to engage myself in additional expenditure, when my main reality problem was how to meet the unavoidable expenses which the state of marriage had brought about! Though, in spite of my desire for knowledge and research, I had temporarily considered a personal analysis superfluous, I was now in a position where I was beginning to wonder whether it was not an absolute necessity, not this time for research purposes, but for therapeutic ones.

My 'cure', far from curing me of all my needs and providing me with the wonderful answer, happiness, seemed to have led me to be in need of a cure. How was I to find it? Well, the answer seemed to be that I could go back to my analyst and resume my daily attendances. It might conceivably lead to something. It had done enough damage so far, perhaps it could not possibly do anything worse, if it is this which is potent enough almost to destroy me, maybe it is potent enough to restore me again. If it cannot do more harm than has already been done, it may do as much good. Though I was very sceptical on that point, it did seem to me a possibility that it might do a little good, at least it might do something to alleviate my internal state of strain and give me some now much-needed support. I could well appreciate the truth that analysis, the need for analysis, like the ego and the need for an ego, is created out of stress and pain, that if we were not frustrated, we would regress instead of evolve.

There had been some little clue in the course of my emotional experiences to the relationship between one affective state and another, and perhaps even a little clue as to the hitherto completely mysterious neuralgic attacks to which I had been subject throughout the greater part of my life of endeavour. The strange thing was that I had noticed during the few months when my love was at a level of unremitting ecstasy, neuralgia had never once so much as suggested its potentiality. It seemed to me, if I thought of it at all, as utterly impossible. But even more curious was the fact that with all this new, very conscious and devastating 'neurosis' which I had recently acquired, the one bogey conspicuous by its absence was neuralgia, and this in spite of my state of worry and strain which I had, on earlier occasions in my life, often thought pre-disposed me to an attack. This time, it seems, I had at least succeeded in substituting one neurosis for another. However, the present one, if not so acutely intolerable, certainly made up for it, or almost made up for it, by being constant and unremitting.

I learnt later that unconscious stresses due to the repression of the instinctual needs can reveal their subterranean presence not only by the periodic eruption of mysterious pains, including intensely acute ones, but even, via automatic physiological channels, in the form of somatic changes and organic diseases, the source of which remains totally unsuspected. Alterations of function resulting from such unconscious stresses lead in due course to alterations of structure. Thus, unless instinct tension is relieved by instinct gratification, it relieves itself, often by changes of function; from functional change we get structural change, and disease. Organic disease is an end-product of processes more morbid than those which cause mental or nervous disorder. An 'unhappy' id (instinct level of the mind), however repressed and unconscious, is an 'unhappy' body. An unhappy ego, such as that implied by the consciousness of worry or conflict and anxiety, is a relatively less, far less, morbid state of affairs. One is more aware of it, but it is just this awareness, this consciousness, of it that makes it superficial and remediable. I had substituted conscious stresses for unconscious stresses; the tensions of a denied and frustrated id had given place to the tensions of a conscious-level worry, a worry which I could conceivably remedy by appropriate behaviour, by activity directed to the real world of economics. I recognised, nevertheless, that there were even less acceptable complications involved in the situation, complications of an emotional nature which affected my subjective relationship to Celia and which might threaten sooner or later the very foundation upon which all this worrysome structure had been built.

CHAPTER XIV

BECOMING AN ANALYST

IT was while I was in the throes of these problems, meditations, worries, and perplexities, that the seeds of the situation which I had sown at the time of emotional ecstasy naturally came to fruition, further to complicate the already overloaded situation. My wife gave birth to a son. I daresay this sort of thing has happened to married couples before my time and yours, but for me it was a particularly complicated emotional situation.

The complicated feelings I was experiencing in connection with all this were due to the normal joy, excitement, exhilaration and delight of having a child, especially a child by this wonderful and attractive girl I had married, trying to break through the uncomfortable, distressing, worrying, anxiety-provoking reality situation as to how on earth I was going to maintain this standard of living, and yet deal with the accumulating debts. I was almost surprised at myself for being able to feel the joys of parenthood while still acutely aware of the horrible reality situation. My wife, as I had expected, turned out to be a wonderful mother, just as she was a wonderful lover. Incidentally, I have always thought that these two qualities go together. The woman who enjoys love, becomes a loving mother, whereas the frigid woman is cold to her children. Celia was delighted to have a baby, and she was as loving and charming as ever, in spite of the accumulating pile of unpaid bills. Under the pressure of economic worries, I then engaged myself in the evenings with a matter to which I had never previously given any application. It was account books. I became an amateur accountant. Accountancy, I may say, was a subject that was anathema to me. I had sat up late one night, working out these figures, and rushed off the next morning to the North London practice, where I had now become almost as busy as I was before the advent of my partner. I had found that morning a little stiffness about my body, and thought it was probably due to an awkward position I had sat in while doing the accounts the previous night, the accounts which had increased my depression. As the day wore on, my bodily discomfort, now assuming the form of abdominal stiffness, gradually increased, and by that afternoon I was walking about, carrying my little bag, distinctly bent because it was painful or well-nigh impossible to straighten myself. I began to think that there was something the matter. There was. I had acute appendicitis.

The chief thing I remember about my emergency appendix operation in St. Thomas's Hospital was how happy I felt—I think now of my appendix girl with the sublime expression on her face—but why should I be so happy? Getting myself warded with appendicitis could not possibly solve any of my problems. I was delighted with the hospital, delighted with the nice, pleasant nurses, delighted with all the attention they gave me, delighted with the visitors who came and sat at the foot of my bed—my mother, my sister, my wife. Probably I mention my wife last because I was used to her now, whereas the others were like visitors that one had lost sight of, visitors from one's native land. I was even pleased with the shy young surgeon who, in the presence of somebody, perhaps my wife, said very abruptly: 'How are you this morning?' I stirred myself a little and said: 'Fine.' 'Good,' he said, and passed on immediately, acutely embarrassed. I would rather he had stopped and talked to me, though I was amused at his shyness. Of course, visitors were not always there, but I always had the nurses, and I thoroughly enjoyed them. I enjoyed being looked after like a baby; I felt utterly spoilt. They joked a little amongst themselves when they made the beds, mine and those around me, and I thought what delightful people they were. A succession of different probationers were put on to do the morning washing or bathing, and I think I fell in love with them all. I remember one was a tall, sinewy girl, obviously from a British public school. She reminded me a little of Margaret, the girl I took through Paris to my sister's chalet in Switzerland. She did her bathing job with such unsmiling, ritualistic seriousity (forgive the neologism—she and her sort could never have invented it) that I almost loved her for her ridiculousness—for she did not seem to be shy. How do we manage, especially in this country, to breed people like this?

It occurred to me what a pity it was that I had not had this experience fifteen years ago, before I came into these wards as surgical dresser or medical clerk. I would have understood the work of the hospital far better than I had ever understood it. I would have appreciated the nursing staff and all the staff, the management, and every bit and piece of surgical and medical attention infinitely better if only I could have had my appendicitis just before the age of twenty, instead of in the thirties. Or would I have been too embarrassed then to be capable of enjoying it, as I was certainly enjoying it now?

After the first week, I was moved into the 'small ward' which had now become vacant. Immediately the whole situation changed. I did not like being in a room alone. The activities in the ward which entertained and intrigued me all day along were not there. I suppose also I was getting better and stronger, for I became restless. By the tenth day, after my stitches had been taken out, I was agitating to get away. The Sister told my wife that I was now like a restless tiger, they had to keep me confined because she felt if I got out of that little ward, there would be no stopping me anywhere. The wise old female treated me with a faintly amused, womanly indulgence. I fancy she was a little bit thrilled at the evident maleness of my restless activity. Anyhow, I did get out of it, in less than a fortnight after the operation. Possibly too soon, for subsequently I was inclined to a period of slight depression lasting some weeks. The conscious mind knows that an operation is designed to help one, to put something that is wrong right again, that it is a kindly, helpful act; on the other hand, the unconscious levels of the mind are quite incapable of appreciating anything so subtle. All they know, and they know it however deep the anaesthetic, is that some interference with their pleasure principle has occurred, a drastic interference, something that caused them pain and mutilation, and continued pain after the mutilation. The unconscious levels appreciate that something dreadful, something terrible, has been done to one, terrible because a little more of this and one would have been annihilated for ever more. Annihilation, death, has been very near indeed; security has been dispelled by this fact. It is as though for all the unconscious knows, the same horror may happen again at any moment, and this time with completely annihilating results. Well, in the light of all this, the unconscious has plenty of grounds to feel apprehensive and depressed. It has been through a bad time. A holiday is the least we can do to reassure it, to tell it that the world is meant to be gratifying, not castrating or annihilating.

Perhaps it was the sojourn at St. Thomas's Hospital that had given me time for reflection and convinced me that whatever else I did or did not do, I had to follow my own individual drive or compulsion. I was a person, I knew, designed by nature for research. I could not stifle the enquiring, question-asking, knowledge-seeking compulsions within my mind, and be happy. They were the compulsions that moved me. It was only in obeying these urges, not in resisting them, that I could be myself. I did not regard myself as *cursed* with this compulsive drive; on the contrary there was so much pleasure in pursuing it and in the fruits, however meagre, which the quest constantly brought, that resigning oneself to this 'compulsive neurosis' was in itself happiness, a happiness that was more characteristic of me than was any other, neurotic or otherwise. I must find myself again. For what shall it profit a man, if he shall gain the whole world, and lose his own soul.

The simplest and easiest move towards that end would be to see my analyst with a view to resuming analysis. As I have said, there now seemed to me more reasons than one for doing so. Previously, the sole reason I could allege was research work. Analysis, I had been told by the President, was the only real training for the purpose of understanding the unconscious mind, one's own, and, for that matter, anyone else's. The essential world of the mind lay hidden from consciousness. It could not, by any other process than personal analysis, be revealed to consciousness because between the unconscious mind and the conscious, there was built up an enormous resistance. You cannot tell people what lies in the unconscious and expect them to believe it. Indeed, the topmost levels of the unconscious, the so-called repressed unconscious, consists solely of a world which has been pushed down there just because the conscious levels of the mind do not like it. That is, in fact, why they repressed it, so they will only be annoyed by any exposition of it in conscious terms. Thus, we cannot know anything below the level of consciousness by any ordinary method or device. It is only through the technique of lessening, reducing or removing the great barrier of resistance between conscious and unconscious, that this intriguing world, absolutely necessary for an understanding of neurotic symptoms, of all symptoms, of symptomatic behaviour, of all behaviour, of anything and everything that is man, can be revealed. Thus, there was no doubt in my mind that my first step towards resuming my researches must be via my own personal analysis. I needed it as an essential preliminary to the understanding of the field of research, the world of the mind, in which I had canalised my compulsive thirst for insight into the nature of things.

In order to do this, it became quite clear to me that I must sell out, I must sell this beautiful house at Mill Hill with its splendid oak tree and all the furnishings it contained. Anyhow, I had never wanted to acquire it, my heart had never been in it, it was against my better judgment that I allowed all this to take place in the first instance. The least I could do now was to cross out my past mistakes. I was surprised at how readily my wife agreed. Maybe she had recognised that I was constituted to be more than a pawn in the biogenic and economic scheme of life; maybe she had some adventurous spirit which was always ready to discard the old and to try something new; maybe she had grown tired of the adventure of launching ourselves into a good-class, conventional mode of living beyond our means; maybe the prospect of remaining *status quo* for twenty years, until the property became our own, was no more congenial to her than it was to me. Anyhow, she readily agreed, and we immediately found a willing, almost overwilling purchaser. Furniture and fittings were all taken at their valuation, and after the settlement with both mortgagors and the furniture stores, we actually discovered that we had lost nothing; in fact, I think we may have been a hundred pounds or so in hand, which we could regard as a re-imbursement, as it were, for a year of struggle.

The feeling of intense relief which I experienced was hardly diluted by regrets at leaving the splendour. I took a last look at the oak tree, and gave a great sigh of relief that I would never need to see it again. What did it stand for? A substitute, some false symbol. It offered me conventional civilisation, a faked-up valuation in place of the real thing that was me. So long as I could see it I dimly realised that I had sold my soul, my heritage—for an oak tree! Twenty years of oak tree would certainly have been too much. My wife found a moderately sized flat in Ormond Terrace on the first floor, with a lovely balcony overlooking Primrose Hill—this was before Ormond Terrace had been converted into a series of little modern flats. My analyst's house was within easy walking distance, which was an added convenience; in fact, the whole situation was infinitely more convenient than

Mill Hill, living at which without a car embarrassed all my work both in North London and at the Tavistock, and would have made attendances at analysis an added complication. Here, on the other hand, it was convenient for everything. I came from my North London practice by bus, visited my analyst, and arrived home for lunch, before proceeding to the afternoon's work at the Tavistock Clinic, or elsewhere. Of course, the enormous advantage above all else was the financial solvency, and the prospect of remaining solvent. On this basis, everything else was practicable. My worry and anxiety had gone, my researches, specifically in the shape of my analysis, had begun again. The year's interval, the year's break from analysis, had taught me something. I felt I had paid pretty heavily for the lesson. Now, at last, I had come back to sanity. Everything was going to be all right again.

At my analysis, I soon took up the threads from where I had left off, the movement started again, and before a week had passed, I was remembering and producing dreams, whereas for the previous year there had been none; perhaps I had been too worried to remember them. Dreams are not to be ignored, particularly in the early stages of analysis. They have been described by Freud as 'the royal road to the unconscious'. There can be no doubt that they should be regarded as emissaries from the unconscious, teaching us, when we have learnt to read their cipher, the precise nature of the repressed complexes, of the emotionally-charged constellations that exist in the deeper and otherwise inaccessible levels of the mind. It is the energy belonging to these complexes which is responsible for our dreams. What makes this of practical, clinical importance is the fact that it is apt to emerge not only in the form of dreams, but also in the form of symptoms and symptomatic behaviour. Indeed, the patterns of energy belonging to these unconscious complexes may be regarded as the source of all our motivations and even of our thoughts and beliefs themselves. Thus it will be seen that the interpretation of dreams can be a very valuable way of learning the nature of the unconscious complexes responsible for them and for symptoms alike, not to mention the springs of our behaviour, beliefs and biases.

At the resumption of my analysis, a series of dreams that impressed me very much may be described as belonging to the 'mother-rescue' variety. I shall record two of them, if only to correct the erroneous impression that may have been created by the one dream I previously mentioned as occurring at the very beginning of my analysis. That dream, the reader may remember, had evidently been stimulated by certain reactions, and transferences to my analyst, a male, and represented my resistance to the negative or inverted aspect of the Oedipus complex. Some of these mother-rescue dreams clearly originated from the positive Oedipus complex, and included hostile attitudes and dealings with the villainous father-image. I cannot adequately convey to the reader how completely alien these revelations appeared to me at the time. I might have been reading fairy tales written by Hans Andersen or Grimm, so dissociated was I, as are we all before analysis, from the unconscious source of everything that is us!

In one of these dreams, I actually saw a magnificent mediaeval castle, and observed the hateful and villainous lord of the castle who appeared to me slightly foreign and certainly capable of the most heinous crimes. I knew that he had a beautiful, flaxen-haired damsel imprisoned therein, and that his intentions towards her were evil to the nth degree. He was alternately striding or loitering about the battlements. The other dream was, of all dreams I have ever had, the most vivid and the most noteworthy on account of its presentation of a chronic emotional characteristic. It is a pity that it had, in contrast to its emotional intensity and vividness, very little conceptual content. Although it was a mother-rescue dream, father does not seem to figure in it at all, or at least not in the remembered portion. It is simply between mother and me. So far as I can remember, it started with the picture of an exquisitely beautiful ballerina, pirouetting upon the railings of a balcony that projected from some extraordinarily high skyscraper. The streets below were full of entranced crowds, all straining their eyes upwards at this enthralling figure. How I could see that she was the quintessence of loveliness from such a distance is, of course, part of the miracle of dreams. She proceeded to perform a series of amazing ballet and acrobatic feats upon this balcony, or rather upon the very railings of it. My heart was in my mouth, I dared not breathe. The intensely emotional tone of the dream was accentuated by the crowd, all similarly spellbound. Suddenly, what might well have been expected, happened. She lost her foothold and came hurtling down to crash in the road, only a few yards from my feet. With bleeding heart, I was at her side in an instant, my whole being just one great solicitude for her succour. I whispered heartfelt words in her ear (she was evidently still conscious in spite of it all!) promising that I would give my very life for her, even to save her from the slightest hurt. Somehow she was on an operating table by now, my arm was round her neck, supporting her lovely head, and I was almost kissing her tenderly as I whispered: 'Fear not; you will feel no pain. I will put everything right.' What is more, I was as good as my word for I had my hypodermic syringe filled and ready, and instantly, with the tenderest love, I introduced the needle and pressed home the injection.

It was after this dream that my analyst, in ribald jest not usually practised by analysts, christened me Aesculapius. Though I had, of course, the usual vague conception of his significance in classical mythology, I rushed home afterwards and looked him up in the *Encyclopaedia Britannica*. The account given is inadequate for it is not mentioned that the coiled serpent which he carries on his staff, evidently as the symbol of his healing instrument, has been adopted as the badge of the Royal Army Medical Corps. Of course, one would not expect any reference to its awful Freudian interpretation. The dream depicts poor mother's (i.e. all women's) 'castration', and the man's natural desire to render succour to the limit (i.e. orgasm) of his power—fortunately in accordance with the pattern of his instinct and its gratification. Thus are all the pains of living healed by love, the woman's missing object restored, in the shape of the child, and life—its pains and their cure—perpetuated.

But dreams are subject to ever-increasing depths of interpretation. On a deeper, more physiological, level this dream is a classic depiction of a sudden loss of tumescence, and identification of the consequent castration-phantasy with the pitiful, heart-rending condition of the opposite sex!

I must resist the temptation to go on relating details of my analysis, though I should perhaps remind the reader that dream interpretation, however intellectually fascinating and deep, does not necessarily convince, or adequately bridge the gap or remove the barrier between the repressed unconscious and consciousness. That is usually achieved only through transference, and analysis of transference.

During the first half of my life a perennial problem had always been the conflict between active living and scholarship, between doing and thinking, between life and research. My difficulty was a compulsion towards both. Throughout the history of man, for example in the Middle Ages in this country, a person usually solved this conflict by choosing one *or* the other. The Schoolmen and the scholars were monks who retreated as completely as possible from the hurly-burly of an active life—and in what unrealistic excursions their meditations involved them and the whole of mankind! In connection with this conflict analytical research has a special position in that its subject of study is specifically the mental processes that accompany the actual experiences of living. Thus it would seem not so incongruous to try to lead an active reality life and at the same time to be engaged upon analysis. In fact, the question might arise as to whether it is at all possible to do one without the other. Nevertheless, difficulties are certain to arise and at times to become insuperable.

It seems that I had gone through such an experience. It seems also that I still considered or hoped that in spite of living an active reality life the emotional and other involvements would not necessarily be too great to enable me to continue to research into psychogenesis, and would in fact give me more real material to research into. I think that this proved largely to be true, in keeping with the argument that if one resists the normal compulsion to live one's life one may easily be diverted into abnormal and neurotic ways of thinking as well as of living.

It was in the spirit of experiencing life, not necessarily devoid of research, that I had elected to plunge into General Practice. It is said that 'Man proposes and God disposes'; I had certainly not consciously or intentionally proposed or planned marriage, the production of a family and all the ensuing complications, emotional, economic and otherwise. But young people commonly feel that it is a good idea to try everything once, and I had not been unduly resistant. It was now my lot in common with less research-minded individuals, to cope with the processes nature inside me had set in motion, in the movement of which I was now thoroughly enmeshed.

After I had been engaged in psychotherapy at the Tavistock Clinic for a few years, I took that room in Harley Street, and had

just begun a tentative introduction to analytical private practice
when my invaluable G.P. partner got married and elected to have
a country Practice of his own. I was forced to shoulder the entire
work of what had now become a very large General Practice, at
first without much economic advantage as it was obligatory to
refund him the value of his capital interest in the business. At the
same time I was already seeing a few psychiatric and analytical
patients in Harley Street.

The obvious course was to engage an assistant to help me with
the General Practice. In those days the professional medical
assistant was not always the best asset that a competitive General
Practice could have. The experiences and adventures which I
encountered with a succession of assistants would themselves
be quite a long story, a little unnecessary to the present
work.

It was about that time that my wife gave birth to her second
child, a girl. Although everything had been under the very best
auspices, including nursing home and gynaecologist, the greatest
imaginable misfortune followed this happy event. Within a few
weeks she was desperately ill. It was in the days before sulphona-
mides, penicillin and the antibiotics, and although every measure
was taken to save her life a protracted tragedy ensued the details of
which I would rather not call to mind and record. My distress was
such that the matron of the Home housed me on the premises
during the later days.

By the time things had quieted down, my analysis was nearly
over and I was able to endure matters with greater fortitude than
hitherto, but nevertheless I was so strongly disinclined to continue
the old way of life, and I had so many debts to settle, that I determined to dispose once and for all of my General Practice and resign
myself to research and specialisation. The selling of such a large
practice at the extraordinarily high market figure then prevailing,
itself involved a great deal of business adventure, and it was some
time before genuine purchasers, two brothers fairly newly qualified,
presented themselves as ready, willing and able to pay the entire
market price of the practice and eager to get it at once in the face
of possible competition. The transactions this time went through
without a hitch. I spent a few months willingly introducing them
and was very glad to have honest and able people to hand over

my patients to in contrast to some of the intelligent scoundrels who had come and gone.

I was now thrown back economically entirely upon my as yet very small psychiatric practice, and though I had more capital behind me than ever before in my life, I realised of course that the process of living on capital is neither a sound one materially nor a very comfortable one psychologically. Nevertheless, I recognised that this was to be my lot until I was sufficiently well established in the specialist world for income to equal expenditure. I had not only my mother to support, but also two lustily-growing infants whose demands I well recognised would increase progressively for some decades.

For many years my concept of economics had been to rely upon dependable income from the General Practice, however small this income might be, to provide me with the necessary security while my psychiatric practice in Harley Street was in its embryo stage. Anxiety had led me to the idea of holding on to the General Practice almost indefinitely until the income from psychiatry had proved itself adequate. But the tragic events following the birth of my daughter had precipitated me into the sudden readjustment which had not been part of my calculations. Though I now had the capital from the practice, I also had three persons dependent on me, and I had burnt my boats regarding General Practice. As it was necessary to support my mother in some degree of civilised comfort, I decided that the best adjustment to the reality situation while I was nursing my specialist practice into an adequate degree of development, and to prevent capital from being frittered away, was to purchase one of the very large houses that were then upon the market, convert it into flats, live in the garden flat myself with my mother and children, and hope that the rent from the other flats in the building would be enough to keep me solvent in the meantime. It was on this account that I bought a large house in Fitzjohn's Avenue and proceeded with this plan. There was no difficulty in filling up one's time between the very lowly-paid work at the Tavistock Clinic, my relatively small but more remunerative and growing psychiatric practice and my analysis and training analysis at the London Clinic of Psycho-Analysis. It was not an unpleasant life. My car would be left each morning at the door of my over-magnificent house, and the rest of the day passed in what was to me the most interesting manner imaginable. The only disquieting thing about this situation was that the monthly bank returns almost regularly showed that I was losing capital at the rate of approximately ten pounds a week, and one knew that this could not go on for ever.

It is usual for a beginner in analysis, or rather in a private analytical practice, to receive his new patients through some senior and established sponsor who has too many applicants to handle himself. A man in this privileged position is in the habit of passing his overflow to his less busy and junior colleagues. In the psycho-analytical and psychotherapeutic circles in which I mixed I was fortunate in receiving patients, not so much from those in the highest position, but through the medium of colleagues and friends. Perhaps I was a little bit senior to most of those at the classes with me and therefore favoured as regards private consultations and private analysis.

Thus my private practice grew at a rate that, though not in any way phenomenal, was gratifyingly steady and progressive. It became increasingly clear, even in those early years, that I would not have to devote so much time to work at institutions, where the remuneration was often nil or negligible, but that the demands of private work would increasingly take up so much of my time that I would have to withdraw some of my hospital and clinical commitments. I may say that the movement in this direction was a sheer necessity if my specialisation projects were going to succeed at all, or even become and remain a practical possibility. For many years one of the difficulties of life remained that of making ends meet, but strangely enough that did not seem to detract from my overweening interest in the scientific aspect of the work, if anything it had the effect merely of increasing my determination to work harder and harder. I was never over-anxious. I read every book on the subject and was so interested in the actual work with my patients that I began, almost involuntarily, as it were, to write little articles based upon my own personal experiences with them. These I published anonymously, partly to help to conceal identities, and partly because I was myself at that period of my life extremely shy of any publicity. I may say that in the course of seven years, I published over a hundred anonymous articles in this way. In the meantime, the Tavistock Clinic had expanded in every respect. A research department had been established, and when the head of this advertised for a piece of original research on clinical material, I gave him my latest article. It happened to be the one entitled 'A Case Diagnosed as Epilepsy'. This brought him post-haste to see me and appeared to create some undue excitement in the Department. It seemed to me it was not research that some people were concerned with, so much as propaganda for the Clinic. I had to confess to him that his hunch was right and that I was, unbeknown, a much practised writer of clinical articles.

Briefly it was the case of a man, who at the age of forty years had suddenly exhibited and continued, a series of epileptiform fits indistinguishable from those of genuine epilepsy. That is to say they were characterised by sudden onset (especially at nights), total loss of consciousness, tonic rigidity and clonic movements, involuntary evacuations of bladder, tongue bitings and other injuries. Nevertheless, some discerning psychiatrist had detected a psychological element, suggested partly by the late age of onset of the fits, and sent the man for treatment. In due course under analysis the patient's rigid mentality gradually gave way, and he got into the habit of producing on the settee intensely highly charged emotional material of an aggressive and hysterial character. At first this was accompanied, during the actual sessions, by an extraordinary physical performance—teeth grinding, face and body contorting, tonic postures and convulsive movements—which could only be described as a major *hysterial* fit, because there was no loss of consciousness accompanying it. Very soon it became obvious that there was a direct relationship between the onset of such a fit and the specific nature of the analytical material. Invariably it was an emergence of the most intense hatred for his deceased father which produced the attack. In the early stages one had only to mention a key-word, such as 'father' or 'murder', for an attack to begin. As one expected the epileptiform fits disappeared entirely and the emotional (hysterical) outbursts, which had taken their place, gradually diminished as the highly charged and previously repressed complexes of childhood and infancy emerged into consciousness.

In those days the *British Medical Journal* was very resistant to psychoanalytical material, and this article led to a quarrel between its two principal editors. One of them was extremely anxious to publish it, and officially accepted it, whereas the other was equally determined that such stuff should not besmirch the Journal's scientific purity. So it went into the *British Journal of Medical Psychology*. Many years later it was re-published in my book *Clinical Psychology*.

It was about this time that I began to receive case after case from the practice of a very eminent psychiatrist and psycho-analyst of the most senior school, and a personal pupil of Freud's. It seemed to me strange, as I had met him on only one or two occasions. The consequence of this was that within three or four weeks, my private practice became full to over-flowing. Looking for an explanation of this experience, I called at his door to thank him. The door was opened by his secretary. She informed me to my surprise that the eminent physician had died a few weeks previously and the reason I was receiving his patients was that she had had verbal instructions from him to send them all to me. She was merely obeying his dying wish. He had bequeathed to me also the greater part of his library. I naturally felt rather frustrated at being unable even to offer him thanks in return. I could hardly have won him by my onymous published works, for at that time I do not think they amounted to more than half a dozen scientific articles. How-ever, my exceeding good fortune proved to be short-lived, for it was about then that the Second World War overtook us. With it there was of course a general exodus from London, and my now full private psychiatric and analytical practice melted away within a few weeks, under the threat of bombing and the beginning of the big air raids.

At the inception of war, I was so convinced that everything would be decided in the air, and that the only unsafe place to be in was under the air (on the ground), that I formed a private theory that the country that was most airborne would be the one to survive. It was on this account that I induced my younger brother to accompany me to the aero-club at Hatfield, and got them to put our names down for instruction in flying. My idea was even at the age of nearly fifty to become a pilot without delay, secretly with an eye on the possibility of becoming an air-fighter! Of course, I had no idea that it would prove not to be a question of being in the air, but a question of the efficiency of the machine, and that that was the only thing which would determine air battles. We are now so air-wise that it seems incredible that anyone could have been so ignorant at that time. Thus it was that although my name was taken and placed on their list for training, it was fortunate for me that the programme of instruction in civil aviation was abandoned by the authorities before it got under way.

CHAPTER XV

THE MENTAL HOSPITAL

THROUGHOUT my psychiatric specialisation there was one branch of the subject in which I felt myself palpably deficient. Although for ordinary analytical purposes one's own personal analysis is the crucial training, nevertheless in the sister-role of psychiatrist, one is periodically confronted with a psychiatric patient sent presumably by a doctor who does not distinguish between the psychiatrist who is mainly engaged in analytical work, and his colleague, the asylum diagnostician. I had throughout felt that my experience in psychiatry proper was insufficient, as I had not had an adequately long training as a resident in a mental hospital.

I felt that this disappearance, or near disappearance, of private analytical practice, presented me with the opportunity I had been looking for. A colleague told me that they were short of medical officers at a very large private mental hospital in London. *How* short they were I had not realised, but when I interviewed the medical superintendent, he was so eager to rope me in that he enthusiastically agreed to every one of my 'conditions', although ordinarily these would have been regarded as quite outrageous. They were, briefly, that if I did the work of a resident medical officer in his mental hospital, I should be allowed to have a private consulting room (as well as my Harley Street one) in the mental hospital itself, and should be at liberty to see private patients and anyone else I chose in this private consulting room, irrespective of my hospital duties. The only condition that he was really eager about was that I should start work immediately—that very day! I arrived for duty the next morning, having evacuated from London my mother and the two children. To my astonishment I found that the medical superintendent, having got my agreement to come, had promptly decamped that very afternoon! The senior medical officer whom he had left behind took over his duties, and I found myself in the position of medical officer to the entire establishment, there being no other. In spite of the bombs, high explosives and incendiaries, regularly raining upon us practically every night, the experiences I had in many months at this establishment

193

were infinitely more pleasant than unpleasant. One soon got to know each of the hundreds of patients in the place, and also acquired a good working knowledge of all the members of the staff. There were at least two psychiatric rounds to be done each day, and usually one at night, when the patients were crowded together in about a dozen enormous underground air-raid shelters. One wore a tin hat and trudged around with a large torch, seeing that everybody was as well and happy as could be expected. During the day-time I had many interesting and amusing experiences as well as the opportunity for a certain amount of psychiatric investigation and learning. One of the routine duties which I disliked most was that of forcible feeding, but fortunately, there were very few cases where this unpleasant job had to be performed and there was some satisfaction in becoming expert at it. The same may be said of the convulsive therapy treatments, particularly in the days before the method of doing them by electric shock had been invented. Naturally it would take a separate book to relate the variety of cases and the intense interest most of them presented.

Patients in a psychiatric hospital are segregated in various wards according to their *behaviour*. I still remember that when I entered the men's convalescent block and found twenty middle-aged gentlemen seated round an enormous covered billiard table, my first impression was that I had entered a Cabinet Meeting. Subsequently I discovered that most of these gentlemen were chronic paranoiacs, and that all of them were certified! Perhaps it was this experience more than any other that made me decide for the rest of my life never to judge anybody's mental equipment by his appearance. One of these members of the 'Cabinet' induced me to accompany him to a secluded part of the building at the end of the corridor, and made me promise that on my daily round I would ascertain that he was still there. When I asked him what he feared, he pointed across the grounds at the laundry chimney, and declared with bated breath that every night a member of the house was carried out there and incinerated.

In the convalescent women's ward, one sat in the lounge before a fire and had tea with the ladies. There I listened to many amusing conversations. One good lady punctuated the tea-party by reading to me various pieces of poetry which she had written since my last visit.

But the most interesting ward was the large one which was referred to simply as Number Eleven. There the women rowdies were segregated. On one occasion I had just passed through the ward and was on my way out when hearing a noise, I looked back and saw the lady of the end bed doing a marvellous pirouette in a most expert manner right along the centre of the ward—stark naked! Of course she was pounced upon by nurses from every direction, and I was somewhat disappointed to miss more of the performance. It turned out that she was a professional ballerina. On another occasion, one of the most severe schizophrenic patients, a large woman, completely mute, stood by her bedside and indicated to me that she had a pain in her mouth. I could see externally that she had a large gum-boil, and decided to investigate it more closely. She opened her mouth on demand and I placed my fingers against her gum to feel if there was palpable pus present. As I turned round after this quick investigation, I saw the matron, who was with me, as white as a sheet and almost about to faint. She had not expected to see my finger intact again. However, the investigation was not so foolish as it looked. I knew well that this was an impulsive aggressor. Indeed, I had seen her tear the headdress and almost the hair from a nurse who came within her reach only a few days previously, and I had been careful to keep my finger from passing between her teeth. Fortunately, not many of the patients were quite so incalculable as this one, though in schizophrenics, impulsive behaviour, dissociated from the rest of the personality, is not uncommon.

One grows accustomed to all sorts of strange behaviour. I remember watching a demure young lady, a doctor's wife, recently admitted, being escorted across a quadrangle by an unsuspecting nurse. Suddenly, without rhyme or reason, the patient clawed viciously at the nurse, narrowly missing her eye, scratching her face and tearing her collar. It happened so swiftly and impulsively, all in a flash, that one could hardly believe one's eyes, for the next second there was the sweet little lady continuing her walk, obviously not even aware that anything *bad* happened. The only explanation for such phenomena is that they are the work of some dissociated part of the personality (hence the name of the illness 'schizophrenia', meaning 'split mind'). Presumably there is some sudden hallucination, perhaps of being herself attacked, upon which the patient (like a dreamer) acts, and knows nothing about it the moment after.

There was another young woman, called Gertrude, obviously not in this world, who spent all her time scribbling interminably on a piece of paper. She was quiet and trouble-free, silent and mute. She took no notice if you spoke to her, however determinedly you tried to intrude, though sometimes she smiled happily at her own thoughts. Then one day I saw Gertrude, in the dining-alcove off the ward, striding backwards and forwards with arms raised, bulging eyes flashing, face contorted in a state of great emotional excitement, shouting incoherent orders to the space around her. She was in a phase of catatonic excitement. The ward sister merely said 'It doesn't last very long.' One of the most curious things about the exhibition was that all the patients around, some of them pushing their way past her, took not the slightest notice of the arresting spectacle.

Then there was the small manic contingent. One has to see a middle-aged lady in a state of acute mania to appreciate the inexhaustability of the human mind and body. Sometimes it is rushing about restlessly, with enormous activity, clumsily doing foolish things and interfering with everybody, morning, noon and night. Of course, exhaustion, and perhaps death, would supervene eventually, after several days or weeks, if sleep were not forced by injection. On account of the exhaustibility of nurses, one good lady had to be put in the padded cell for short periods, or until an injection could be got ready. She invariably tore off every stitch of her clothing. It was very hot weather, and when the cell door was opened on my round there was a general rush of over-clad nurses to cover her nakedness. I wondered which was madder! While I was at the hospital, we admitted one case of so-called Religious Mania, a florid, pyknic (fat and tubby) lady of fifty, who sang psalms incessantly, interrupting herself only momentarily to ask me if I had been saved.

The other ward full of very sick ladies, namely, depressive, potential suicides was equally well staffed with nurses, but a large number of wards in a mental hospital such as this can often be left with very little supervision. Most of the inmates are extremely well-behaved and almost calculable. In fact, there was one lady in the hospital who was there for three weeks at her own request.

She had, many years previously, been an ordinary inmate, and, having obtained her discharge, returned regularly every year for her three weeks' summer vacation as she felt so attached to the place. She, like many others, would go out daily on parole and return at the appointed hour for her evening meal, for her chat in one of the lounges, and her bed. I tried a tentative analysis with this patient and soon discovered that she was still a little too hypomanic for the process to be continuable with complete safety.

Although one's experience in this establishment was most rewarding as a re-introduction to the sort of case that one does not often encounter in one's analytical private practice, the nightly bombing experiences created an interlude to my scientific work which became increasingly hard to bear. During the time I was there, we had half a dozen high explosives land on the premises, which covered ten acres, and over three hundred incendiary bombs. I became quite accustomed to running about with bags of sand to put out incendiaries. This was fortunately before the explosive incendiaries were invented. The number of times one pulled out of bed people who had been covered with falling debris was quite memorable. Nevertheless, there were surprisingly few real casualties that had to be sent to hospital. I have a clear recollection of standing in the rafters of the Nurses' Home, a building which actually caught on fire, using a hose from that point of vantage to put out the burning floors below. In these roles I certainly did not feel that I was in my appropriate milieu. However, the air raids grew less, and finally faded out. More people were coming to my private consulting rooms. As numbers increased, I found that I could not handle the private work while I was half isolated in this mental hospital, and therefore, when two new medical officers were recruited, I returned exclusively to my practice in Harley Street, again with an almost full house.

A curious personal experience is that, although my nerves stood up tolerably well to those air-raid experiences, when, after a few years of no air raids, the flying bombs began to operate, although infinitely less intensive, I found I could stand them less well. My theory is that in the latent period of about two years between the first experience and its relatively minor successor, certain unseen psychological movements had taken place, which left some mark, like an old wound, which was too sensitive to stand the irritation of restimulation. I feel that this supports my contention, which I base on actual clinical experience, that once a person has suffered anything in the nature of a war trauma (shell-shock), even if it was twenty years or more previously, he should never again be allowed to face battle conditions. I think that, whether he has been analysed or not, something has been done to the mind which makes it tend to break down again if the traumatic experience is repeated, even in a relatively minor form.

As the war receded, my psychotherapeutic practice in Harley Street developed into a very full occupation. There was no general practice now and the pressure of private work grew to such a degree that it claimed more and more of my time, so that public engagements had to give place to it. I was soon in the throes of an occupation which, on account of its enormous time-absorbing qualities, made any and every other interest in life nearly impossible. Patients who came for an interview were commonly eager to begin treatment as soon as possible. Indeed, those who were not so keen were unlikely to turn up for treatment at all, or if they did come, would probably have too much resistance to produce results. The majority could not brook delay, and so one's day tended to become over-crowded, for the type of work was one which could not be done hurriedly, or with any time-saving attempt. The nature of the work precluded the possibility of rapid consultations, and certainly precluded any possibility of skimping the time of sessions. Consultations had to be given at least one hour, sometimes one-and-a-half or two hours. Treatment, involving as it did the essential principle of relaxation, could not be scheduled at less than fifty minutes a session. The result was that intervals for meals and for evening reading or recreation became shorter and shorter, and it was only with difficulty that one safeguarded a minimum of time for oneself. I found my life developing into a daily routine of psychotherapy from about nine in the morning to very nearly nine at night. Nevertheless, it would be quite mis-leading to give the impression that this was an arduous task or a dull and boring way to live one's life. The truth is very much to the contrary. Indeed, sitting in a chair, life is brought to one in fairly large substantial slices, and with infinite variety.

There are many cases in which the results achieved appear to be much less than they actually are, but occasionally one gets a case when the reverse holds good and the *apparent* results of therapy far exceed the true degree of amelioration. Such a case was that of the French woman who had spent two years in bed guarded by a day-nurse and a night-nurse, and attended by a fashionable practitioner, who wore white spats, and who treated her, according to her report, with no less than sixteen different coloured pills in the twenty-four hours. All she had achieved in the time was two 'suicide' attempts, one involving the breaking of a window and the other the cutting of her wrists in the bath. At first she came in a private car with an attendant. After three months she came by taxi. After another three months she came by bus and finally she came on foot, through the Park—running. She and I will both remember the occasion, fairly early in her treatment, when a flying bomb cut-out overhead and she leapt from the settee and pinned me in a corner of the room, covering my precious person with her body and her out-stretched arms, and this despite the fact that we were on a perfectly formal, professional relationship. This impulsive act was subsequently analysed as a demonstration that, given the opportunity, her incestuous desires outweighted her self-preservative instincts! In due course this hysterical invalid actually got a job, a hard-working job. It was connected with the B.B.C. French broadcasts. She then, while still under analysis, took the full training for an officer in the French Women's Army, carried out of the labour wards the weaker sisters who fainted at confinements, and actually embarked for the landing beaches in Normandy on D.12 day, as a full-blown woman officer of the French Auxiliary Service. Subsequently she was mentioned in despatches for her excellent work in charge of a Displaced Person's Camp over forty thousand strong. She ruled the most turbulent, including Russian ex-convicts, with a rod of iron, as she had previously ruled her husband and attendants. But in spite of this commendable display of sublimated energy, sustained for the incredible period of eighteen months, she eventually ran true to form. She developed an incredibly acute attack of abdominal crisis at the characteristic hour of two in the morning and had to appropriate the personal aeroplane of the Army Corps Commander for an immediate night flight to Paris and an emergency appendicectomy. Of course, after that, she made an uninterrupted recovery—why shouldn't she?—and I dare say she has since proceeded from crisis to crisis with every satisfaction except that of adequate psychosexual orgasm. That is why I do not regard her as a cure. She is every bit as ill as was Florence Nightingale at her best.

The difference between the type of life I now found myself leading, and that which I led in general practice, is not easy to describe in a few paragraphs. As in most of our daily occupations, the life of general practice means that a good deal of time is spent, not so much in thinking as in moving around from one place to another, and from one person to another. One rarely has adequate time to devote to any particular individual. In the industrial class of general practice one can listen, perhaps impatiently, for at the most ten minutes, and then have recourse to the time-saving devices of stethoscope, examination and, if required, hospitalisation. On the other hand, in analytical practice there is no such wastage of one's activities. One not only has time for thought, but there is little distraction or interruption in the process of thinking and listening. When I was attending my (interrupted) Membership course at one of our London teaching hospitals, I remember a Senior Physician telling the students not to rush into physical examination of patients. He said: 'The extent of the experience of a good physician may be calculated by the ratio of the time he spends listening to the patient's complaints as compared with the time he spends in performing his physical examination. The student tends to rush straight into the examination, palpating, percussing, auscultating (stethoscope), and all the other paraphernalia of physical examination, whereas the experienced physician, listening long and carefully, may often find that the physical examination, if not superfluous, is at the most merely confirmatory of what he has already gathered from listening to the symptomatology.' One may add that in general practice such instruments as the stethoscope are often, if one must confess the truth, chiefly a time-saving device to cut short the patient's conversation, to impress him favourably, and to enable one to get away expeditely! In a psychiatrist and, more particularly, in an analytical practice on the other hand, this ratio of listening to examination reaches its logical extreme. One listens and thinks all the time, and probably does not perform any physical examination at all. If physical examination is advisable, and has not already been done by a physician, it is often relegated to one. In actual practice one commonly finds that by the time the patient has reached the psychiatrist, he has had a surfeit of doctors and of physical examinations of every description, including very often X-rays, laboratory tests and, saddest of all, occasionally unnecessary surgical interference; whereas the experienced psychiatrist, listening to him for one hour, could have predicted with absolute certainty that there was no organic disease to X-ray or to operate upon. The unfortunate patient had not met a psychiatrist or any sufficiently understanding person who was able to listen thoughtfully for as long as that, and who was knowledge-able and experienced enough to read between the lines while he listened. In fairness I should add that there are many general practitioners who are most experienced at this sort of diagnosis— after all, eighty-five per cent of their patients are neurotic—but often they have not the time and they may not have the confidence to avoid the radiologist and the surgeon.

The professional life of a psychiatrist, particularly an analyst, is to me more satisfying than that of a general practitioner. To most people the latter occupation would be preferred, for most people have to find some outlet or relief for their anxiety. This is commonly achieved by rapid changes of occupation and some-times by what may be called hopping about like a cat on hot bricks from one superficiality to another. The analyst on the other hand has had to be analysed out of his anxiety, and with it the need to relieve his tensions by a succession of rapid changes. His psychology must be that of a desire to go more deeply into things, and his sorrow is that despite all his patience and resource, he can rarely succeed in going quite deeply enough. It is first causes even more than mechanism which he is seeking.

Nevertheless, I must admit that I found the varied and catholic interest of general practice limitless, stimulating and absorbingly interesting. Perhaps it was the best occupation in one's younger days, when energy had to be expended and one was not yet attuned to the relatively steady though slow march of deeper mental investigation. General practice invariably means the expenditure of physical, muscular energy, whereas this is almost excluded from an analytical, psychiatric practice. In both practices I think people and their psychology is, or becomes, the main focus of interest, whether the general practitioner knows it or not. Nowadays he is recognising it more and more. But the difference is that in an analytical practice, you can settle down and satisfy this interest, whereas in general practice it is constantly being frustrated. The average general practitioner certainly has not time to listen for an hour a day to each patient.

CHAPTER XVI

THE PATIENTS

THERE are various misconceptions in the public mind regarding the type of person who comes to a psychiatrist or analyst. Admittedly persons who are seriously ill mentally do come, more especially do they come to the non-analytical psychiatrist. So far as the analyst is concerned, practically all his patients, with the exception of a very occasional consultation, are far from being of the type one associates with mental hospitals. The popular conception is that the analyst's clientele consists largely of peculiar, foolish or simple minded persons: the rich pampered woman, the egocentric who wants to talk about herself. Or if not of these of something even worse, such as sexual perverts, homosexuals, sadists, delinquents, misfits, oddities or more or less brainless idiots. Nothing could be further from the truth.

The truth is that life for every living creature is a battle against frustration—not so much external frustrations as internal frustrations—intra-psychic frustrations. In *homo sapiens* these have been planted there largely by the influence of kind mothers and fathers and successive mentors, teachers, civilisation and the particular culture or mythology in which we live. The modifications which such forces have instigated have been integrated into the growing mind to form a force (called the super-ego), which originally served to check the inherited instinct forces. This battle between instinct that presses for relief of tension, and introjected parent equivalents that inhibit and frustrate this relief, is the classical variety of mental *conflict* which is responsible for the stress and strain within the mind. These stresses and strains, the fruits of conflict, do not always break out and reveal themselves in the form of symptoms, neurotic, psychotic, or physical. They may remain as a painful or intolerable state of stress. In some cases they may not even be *felt*. They may be repressed from consciousness and work their way out as visceral disturbances such as palpitations of the heart, gastric disfunctions, leading to gastric ulcer, rheumatism, diabetes, asthma and a host of others.

The greater part of the battle of frustration is unseen, and so also are the casualties, but casualties there are in abundance—all the time, mental and physical casualties. Indeed, all the ills from which man suffers, from unconscious and invisible internal stresses to major mental and physical illness—and death, not excluding his mass destruction by himself—are to my mind all rightly regarded as casualties of his battle, his struggle against frustrations within him and without. His ego or his will-power is often no more than a helpless spectator, and sometimes not even that, of the movement of forces which may even destroy him from within—and from without.

Now the people who come to an analyst are usually those who are bright enough to sense something of the distress which they are suffering, whether or not this distress shows itself in palpable symptoms. If we read the history of the world, particularly the very early history, and anthropology, even the blindest among us may recognise that there has long been an illness of the world at large. It is hardly logical to assume that there *was* an illness, as for instance in the era of human sacrifice and the burnings of heretics and witches, and that there is no illness at the present day. Indeed, some intelligent observers have come to the conclusion that the illness increases with civilisation and culture. If it is true that we live in such an ill world, surely we will have to be correspondingly ill in order to endure it. Biology teaches us that after all we are only animals in clothes trying painfully to adapt ourselves to captivity, harness and psychological harness.

Anxiety provoking alarums produce physiological reactions appropriate to our original jungle activities of fight or flight, but the stockbroker's or business man's action is limited merely to answering the telephone. So it is not surprising if the sugar released in his blood-stream for sustained muscular instinctual activity contributes to glycosuria or diabetes and the nervous tension to symptoms of an anxiety state. What in a past age would have been appropriate aggressive reaction necessary for survival, must now be inhibited or sublimated to such a degree that it may well be the potentially most healthy person who is the most prone to internal tensions and duodenal ulcers. There are, of course exceptions to this rule. For instance, the American General who is reported to have snarled at his medical officer: 'I don't get Duodenal Ulcers, I *give* them'! And my apparently normal, though rather forceful, patient who bellowed at me the other day: 'I have got bags of energy that I cannot use or that you tell me I cannot use. I am not a squirt like you.' (Incidentally I should mention here that one of the essential qualifications of an analyst is that he must be able to endure, even encourage, *unlimited* vituperative attacks with absolute equanimity. This he can do because his role is that of a scientist investigating the source of emotional explosions, not that of an emotionally driven person relieving his tensions by throwing bombs himself). My patient continued to shout at me: 'All people with my energy blow off, from Churchill downwards. Blowing off is the only relief I can get and that is not enough'. I said to him: 'Perhaps you are trying to blow your frustrating ego out of existence!' Of course, those who 'succeed' in performing such a psychic operation are those who become psychotics. The frustration in this world, against which this patient was raving, is perhaps that none of us can find an adequate outlet for aggressive impulses. It is on this account that we have to be trained from infancy to harness such impulses and must hope to sublimate them. No doubt there are many interesting aspects of this sort of frustration. If we can suppress aggressive instincts, or sublimate them, the result is civilisation. If all we can do is to repress them, the result may be illness, neurotic or physical, Perhaps we do all these things; also perhaps we combine with one another in order to overcome the frustration of these instincts, and so find a way of liberating them in an organised form. That is the psychological basis of war. The illness of the world takes manifold forms. Some can adapt themselves to such a situation, others feel internal stress or strain in endeavouring to do so. It is more likely that we all have more stress than we admit or even know about.

Generally speaking, it takes an intelligent person to recognise not only that he has intolerable stresses, but also that there is a profession which endeavours to understand these stresses, to bring them to consciousness and to co-operate with the sufferer in endeavouring to find a way of dealing with them. A profession which endeavours to do this without necessarily enlisting a system of unfounded beliefs or illusions, magic and nonsense, to aid the process. Sufferers with such a degree of appreciation and insight are often people who have been most successful in the battle of life. In short, the people who come to an analyst are, generally speaking, far from being failures in the ordinary sense of the word, they are often people who have had the greatest outward success in business and professional life, and have only then learnt the bitter truth that it has not adequately relieved their inner state of distress. And they are often people with an unusual degree of energy, perhaps with what Edgar Allan Poe termed 'the fever called "Living" '. If one's internal energy is superabundant, one's task in finding a satisfactory expression of it within the structure of society may present far greater difficulties than in cases where the 'fever called "Living" ' has received cold douches until it has become afebrile, subnormal and apparently non-existent.

Several more or less appropriate examples of patients inflicted with this superabundant energy, often anxiety-driven, crowd upon my mind. There is the case of the shop assistant who saved all his money, worked all the time and played not at all, who became manager, who bought the lease of the premises opposite and opened up in opposition, who subsequently established a chain of shops at cut-prices up and down the country, and who reaped as his reward chronic indigestion and a nervous breakdown. There is the case of the boy whose father went bankrupt and who at the age of fifteen had to find work as a grocer's assistant, who fell out with his employer and took to a barrow, then to a cart and horse, then to several carts and horses, then to stable accommodation for them, then to more stables and to buildings and houses. He is now the proprietor of dozens of companies all over the world, necessitating bi-weekly flights across the Atlantic. The fruits of his incredible success? For several years his overriding wish was that the plane should have a trap-door through which he could *jump* into the Atlantic. To correct a misconception, I must here affirm that the numbers of my male clientele exceed the female in the proportion of three to one.

I have reason to believe that we are all suffering from the same stresses for which my patients come for psychotherapeutic help. Some people are more sensitive and are more disturbed or distressed by frustration than are others, and some are intelligent enough to be driven to seek atl east an explanation in the hope that with understanding they may be in a better position to help themselves.

The battle in the mind can be described as a battle in which energy at an instinctual level endeavours to force its way out through the executive channels of the mind while the resistances of the super-ego and ego oppose its behaviouristic emergence. This latter group of repressing forces may be sufficiently powerful to keep a person from conscious appreciation that there is something there wanting to come out. Repression may be at work, leaving an individual apparently free to deal with what he has learnt to regard as the realities of life. This position of stability will however not render him immune from the effects of the unknown forces deep within the unconscious levels of his mind. They may still operate at an unconscious level and even at a physiological level in the form of organic disturbances such as functional disabilities and even chemical ones. Functional disorders can in time lead to organic changes, and thus all the illnesses to which man is heir can manifest themselves while the sufferer's ego is completely innocent of their source. Here I am referring to the world of medicine proper, and also of surgery.

I have a very disturbed patient who is never tired of telling me that, however ill, mad, bad and sad, I consider him to be, *his* illness is merely mental, whereas I ought to see his brothers and his father and his father's brothers. Every one of them, he says, has a slit down the middle of his belly! He is referring to the familial disease of gastric or duodenal ulcer for which they have each been surgically opened up. He attributes *his* freedom from this disaster to his relatively trivial mental symptoms whereby he discharges his aggressive tensions outwardly (so that others get the tension!), instead of, like his male relations, bottling them up inside to cause duodenal ulcers and surgical operations.

People who present themselves for analysis are on the whole less completely fortified against all conscious sense of their deeper tensions and internal disturbances, than are the majority of those who suffer exclusively from physical, organic, medical and surgical illnesses. They are more or less aware of impulses and drives inside them which create uncomfortable tensions unless they can find some more or less appropriate outlet with which to discharge this psychogenic energy. Extraordinary amounts of energy clamouring for discharge are obviously not necessarily a bad thing for the individual, and certainly not necessarily bad for the community. Indeed it has been said with some justification that 'all great people are neurotic', though I feel it might be more truthful to say that all great people are potentially neurotic; in other words, if they can find an outlet for their nervous energy sufficiently appropriate to earn them greatness, they can be more accurately assessed as great than as neurotic. But when they are frustrated from finding such an outlet, then the energy can only relieve itself in less appropriate ways, including perhaps symptomatic expressions which are regarded as neurotic, psychotic or characterological.

For instance, it has been said of all great authors that they would never have produced their writings had there not been something in them pressing for expression, and very often that something has been very highly charged emotionally. One thinks of people like the Brontë sisters, Dickens, Scott, Chatterton, Oscar Wilde, and perhaps all great writers without exception. Florence Nightingale has been alleged to have had something burning inside her (perhaps symbolised by the proverbial lamp!) which obtained its outlet in the activities responsible for her greatness, at the expense of the peace of mind of Cabinet ministers, government, and populace. In fact we may say she created emotional disturbances or hysteria in all the otherwise placid minds around her. When, in the latter part of her life, she could no longer do this, her emotional fire expended itself in what has been called 'frank, screaming hysteria'. In other words, these emotional fires within can create greatness as well as intolerable internal discomforts, psychotic, neurotic, and organic disturbances.

The sort of person who presents himself to a psychiatrist is one who has become aware of a considerable degree of internal discomfort, whether or not some involuntary or symptomatic expression of this discomfort which he dissociates from himself (his ego), has intruded itself upon his attention. In other words, he may present himself without a single describable symptom at one end of the scale, or with a poly-symptomatology of almost every conceivable organic physical, nervous and mental disturbance at the other end of the scale.

The commonest of all symptoms which causes a person to present himself for therapy is the feeling of *Anxiety*. This is substantially analogous to fear, and if it reaches any degree of intensity is one of the most uncomfortable sensations and perhaps the most difficult to endure. Indeed, it is so difficult to endure beyond a certain point, that the psyche endeavours automatically and involuntarily to reduce it by diverting the energy or tension of Anxiety along an infinite variety of channels, visceral, organic and psychic, in an endeavour to get rid of it somehow. Thus severe anxiety cases commonly present themselves with a symptom or a multitude of symptoms, indeed under this heading might be included the entire medical, surgical, psychoneurotic and psychotic lists of symptomatology. The task of analysis is to discover the source of the Anxiety, which in itself is the source of the multiple symptomatology.

An over-simplification would be to regard the Anxiety as the reaction of the ego to unconscious instinct-based energy that is threatening to overthrow the repressing and controlling forces. Thus the individual's ego reaction is as though he were about to be thrown out of control and overwhelmed by some force which he does not identify as himself. Nevertheless, this is the simple truth in a large proportion of Anxiety States. A typical case is that of the married woman who presents herself with some early anxiety symptom such as dizziness or palpitation of the heart. One discovers that for the past five years or so, perhaps since the birth of her last child, she has been subjected by her husband to the contraceptive practice of *coitus interruptus* (withdrawal), At first she suffered merely the transient feelings of disappointment, of being 'left in mid-air'. But she will tell you it did not matter very much, because she soon reached her present happy state of not being interested in sex anyhow, or having practically no feelings about it or about the practice of it. This was followed by an actual distaste of everything connected with 'making love'. Unfortunately this distaste in due course extended to some inexplicable dislike of her husband, towards whom she had previously been quite warm-hearted. But she will tell you all this has nothing to do with her symptoms for she has become quite frigid and almost anaesthetic sexually. She does not now find it too difficult to put up with her husband's attentions, because he is considerate and 'does not trouble her very much'. 'Yes', it was after a few years of sexual frigidity or anaesthesia

o

that she got this outcrop of nervous troubles—which proves that
sex had nothing to do with it!

Within this category of Anxiety State are also the cases of
engaged couples who have been subjecting each other to a good
deal of excitement without a proportionate amount of relief.
Indeed I believe the trouble was once called 'the nervous illness
of engaged couples'! On analytical investigation of the sufferer
and the symptoms, the impression is sometimes gained that he or
she is, as it were, on the verge of something very like a displaced
orgasm. It is a state of chronic excitement or impending crisis—
anxiety crisis; the very antithesis of sexual crisis. Indeed it would
appear that the ego is in a perpetual state of fright as though
something might occur which it will be unable to control. And, sure
enough, all sorts of things do occur which it is unable to control,
such as giddiness and floating sensations in the head and indescribable feelings in any part of the body. It is often more correct to
regard current sexual frustrations as precipitating causes super-
imposed upon a more deep-seated aetiology. Nevertheless, it is
usually true to say that the nervous breakdown would not have
occurred without them.   .

I have suggested that the above may be an over-simplification
of the psychology of anxiety, because for one thing it depends
upon mental structure, that is to say, on a degree of psychic
development in which different structural levels of the mind can be
differentiated, such as instinct levels, and super-ego and ego
levels. Freud endeavoured to elucidate at least three hypotheses
of anxiety. His first was that ungratified libido was directly
transformed into anxiety, his second, also in keeping with what
I have been saying, was that anxiety arose from the ego being
afraid of not being able to control instinct pressure; the third
which can be regarded as a sub-variety, arises in the ego from
a feeling that it has incurred the disapproval of the super-ego.
This is the feeling of guilt (a form of anxiety) and is obviously
an intrapsychic equivalent of the child's fear of having displeased
the parents.

In more recent times some pyschoanalysts have stressed that
anxiety can exist prior to structural development of the psyche,
and that it can be attributable to the struggle between life instincts
and death instincts on the lowest instinctual plane. An unpublished

theory of mine is that the 'guilt' (above mentioned) is a structural equivalent of this, the 'death' instincts (destruction, aggression, etc.) having gone over to the construction of the super-ego. Hence guilt feelings can lead to self-destruction (suicide). A theory which I have published and stressed is that anxiety arises whenever there is frustration of the gratification-aim of an instinctual impulse.* The living organism itself naturally reacts as though its life is being threatened, as indeed may well be the case. If we cannot get enough air we feel anxiety, and our life *is* being threatened. What complicates the picture is the fact that instinct-gratification can be frustrated from within as well as from without.

In contradistinction to the view of some psychologists, my theory is that whenever unrelieved tension arises within the organism, even in an amoeba (e.g. causing cell division), this tension is identical with what we know on a higher plane as anxiety. I am here referring to a very basic symptom, perhaps the basis of all symptoms, and indeed to its most basic and simplified form. In practice, the condition has usually become very much more complicated in the psyche of the person who presents himself for treatment. Whatever basic tensions he is suffering within, they have usually attempted to relieve themselves in a variety of symptoms, visceral or behaviouristic, which are interfering with his happiness and with his ego–syntonic and conscious purpose in life. For instance, he may be so repressed that he is unable to hold his own in relation to other people's aggressive and emotional expressions of themselves at his expense. This repression can be due to anxiety reaction regarding his own aggressive and emotional potentialities. At the opposite end of the scale, he may be unable adequately to control expressions of aggressive or emotional pressure within himself, and may be subject to outbursts of an hysterical nature which disturb his peace of mind and that of others and commonly give rise to feelings of anxiety in connection with them, or seriously handicap his social and business life. We all know that the over-shy or timid person feels uncomfortable in society and is therefore prone to eschew it and become a recluse. What we do not so readily appreciate is that the comparatively uncommon vitriolic aggressive person is liable to do the same. A patient said to me 'My sister stammers

* "The Fundamental Nature of Anxiety"—*Brit. Jnl. Medical Psychology*—1951.

in company; I shout, and make other people stammer. If I held my reactions in, I'd become all tense and stammer myself like she does'. Neither of them are happy or comfortable with people, and therefore they tend to be lonely.

It is not unusual in some cases for the situation of internal tension or anxiety to have progressed beyond this point, so that the individual becomes a victim of various morbid fears, commonly regarding his own health. He may have periodic or chronic scares in connection with his physical condition, imagining he has some terrible disease such as cancer. A patient whose Anxiety State has developed to this state of hypochondria generally suffers much more from his hypothetical cancer than many people do from the actual physical disease.

I had a man patient in the later thirties who periodically, or almost continuously, suffered very acutely from some hypochondriacal illusion or delusion. His favourite 'disease' was cancer, perhaps the most popular of all in this sort of scare. First he got it in his tongue, (actually he had a tooth which irritated one side of his tongue, and he could not get it out of his head that it was the beginning of tongue cancer), subsequently this was cured, but within two weeks the slight pain which he had in his chest definitely suggested to him that he had cancer of the lung. He went to his doctor, and nothing would satisfy him short of a physical examination and X-ray. Once this was cleared up he felt much better, but his happy state lasted for less than two weeks. He then got an abdominal pain, which again convinced him that he had cancer, this time in the stomach. No sooner was this investigated, and the illusion dispelled, than he had a peculiar feeling in his anus, which he felt certain was cancer of the rectum. The poor doctor again had to subject this patient to a physical examination. And so it went on, month in and month out. When cancer had a temporary rest, he then scratched his finger, and was convinced that tetanus would be the result. Indeed, he experienced a little stiffness of his jaws, 'proving' that the dread disease was coming on. He had to go to his doctor again, and again nothing would satisfy him but the inappropriate physical remedies, anti-tetanic serum, etc. An interesting point about this case, and his tetanus phobia, was that while he feared tetanus so much, and took every precaution against scratching or cutting himself in any way, nevertheless, or perhaps on this very account, he was constantly at this period, having little accidents which set the thing ablaze. He even managed to scratch the knuckle of one of his fingers against a screw on my consulting-room door. The anxieties consequent upon this preoccupied him for several weeks.

A particularly interesting symptom of this advanced case of Anxiety was that when hypochondriacal illusions faded, he suddenly discovered that he was in some way connected by marriage with the Jewish fraternity, and in consequence of this very tenuous connection, he felt sure that he would one day be beaten up by anti-Semitic rioters. The interesting point here is that the 'bad object', (as we call it in psychology), when it was not internal, and part of his body, became external and part of the social body. To cure such a case, analysis has to go right back to a very early period of a patient's life, or psychic development. He is, at that stage of life, preoccupied with part-objects, good and bad. The bad ones happen to have been largely introjected and, in subsequent life have developed into a fear of these internal destructive agents.

It is from such psychic conditions as these, whether or not they develop into definite phobias, that many cases of drug addiction arise, including the fairly general one of excessive alcohol consumption. Incidentally, recourse to such palliatives, like every movement away from the hidden source of the trouble, tends to make therapy more difficult. The tension of unrelieved anxiety, if it has not found adequate safety-valves in the form of symptoms, can be responsible for sudden losses of consciousness, fuges, black-outs, and in my opinion, epilepsy, or something very like it. A more chronic or continuous form which the fear of instinctual relief may assume is that of obsessional neurosis which often shows itself in symbolical form as a series of more or less systematic precautions against involuntary reliefs. Of course, such measures are commonly accompanied by an admixture of the very thing they are taking precautions against. Even accidents can be an admixture of self-destroying or self-damaging impulses combined with excessive and inappropriate precautions against them.

A very distressing case I had was that of a man who identified his excrement (to a greater degree than is common amongst us all)

with some poisonous or destructive, germ-ridden agent, which had
to be taken precautions against, to a fantastically obsessive extent.
When he touched any part of his trousers, even the braces, he had
to go and wash his hands, usually several times. When he took a
bath, he had to have a succession of baths, but even then he felt
that the poisonous agent was only diluted and never completely
eradicated. He was constantly putting on several layers of clean
underpants. Now the curious thing about all these precautions was
that in spite of them, or perhaps because of them, this poor man
was constantly suffering from occasional little soilings of these
very underpants (as though his id was rebelling against the
tyranny) and in consequence working himself up into frenzies of
anxiety. It may be appreciated that normal sexual life could not
so much as get an innings.

A certain proportion of people who present themselves for
treatment are victims of cyclothymic disorders. That is to say,
like most of us, they are subject to alternating phases of depression
and elation, only in their case the swing of the pendulum may
exceed its normal range. I am not referring specifically to manic-
depressive psychoses, in which the degree of activity and elation
may be quite intolerable to everybody, and in which the degree
of depression amounts to dangerous and suicidal melancholia,
but rather to a condition of cyclothymia that deviates from the
normal only to a degree which commonly eludes recognition, both
by the sufferer and by those around him. If the individual is
merely slightly hypomanic, he is unlikely to appear for treatment,
but may on the contrary achieve a great deal of material success
and will certainly achieve a great deal of self-satisfaction. It
is probably only his wife and family who will complain of the
shallowness of his emotional life. If, on the other hand, it is
his depressive phases which are more protracted or severe, everything is possible from suicide to drink or electric convulsive
therapy. It is only if he presents himself to a psychiatrist that
diagnosis is likely to be established.

Such a case was that of an American doctor who came to see
me, brought by his wife, because he had lately taken to despairing
about his future, and had tried to cure his sufferings by excessive
whisky-drinking. It transpired that he had had practically the
opposite sort of temperament until the last two months. He had,

I was told, always been rather a happy person, and if anything, over-confident about himself and his future. This recent realisation of the insecurity of his position was literally driving him to drink. On investigation, it transpired that nine years ago he had been the victim of a similar attack, under very different circumstances. When one enquired further back into his life, one found that some eleven years before that, again there had been a phase of depression and despair. This history had been ignored until I drew attention to it. I was relieved to find that these phases usually lasted only about four months. On this basis, one could diagnose this man as a mild case of manic-depressive trouble. The diagnosis was important in so far as it enabled one to reassure the family that in all probability the present was just one of the recurrent phases of depression, which would disappear in the same way that the previous phases had disappeared, and that in all probability he would regain his customary good spirits, or hypomanic condition. Amongst such cases are those in which a severe bout of depression may lead to suicide.

A large proportion of people and their relatives, acquaintances and friends are the victims of a psychopathic personality, commonly with some paranoid (or slightly delusional) admixture.

The difficulties that some wives experience from their husbands, and the difficulties that some husbands experience from their wives, are sometimes due to their having married what the psychiatrist would call a slightly psychopathic personality. There is every degree of such troubles, some of which are almost impossible for anyone closely associated with the person, to tolerate. Social and legal attitudes seem to indicate a lack of appreciation of these facts and to be as incompetent to deal with them as are the victim or victims. One hears of married couples still sleeping in the same double bed though for years they have so loathed each other that they have balanced themselves on opposite edges of the mattress. Surely such people are lacking in capacity for adjustment. One thinks that they might at least have fallen out of the bed! These persons rarely come to the psychotherapist unless their particular pyschopathic trend is causing them insuperable discomforts and sufferings with which they find themselves unable to cope.

People with abnormal sexual tendencies, other than impotence and frigidity, are not likely to seek psychiatric aid on their own account, though they do occasionally do so. More commonly they find some more or less gratifying adjustment in real life. They are more likely to seek psychotherapy if their mental constitution is such that they are extremely resistant to their particular emotional trend, or feel a great degree of anxiety in consequence of it.

These peculiarities of psychosexual pattern are not restricted to stupid people by any means. Once upon a time I had a professor from one of the provincial universities, who, in the course of his analysis, revealed that he was in the habit periodically of visiting a lady friend in a distant part of the town, in whose flat the pair of them enacted the most extraordinary drama. When he gave his special knock, she would open her flat door, standing concealed behind it; he would walk straight through, with his suitcase, into the bathroom. There he would open his suitcase, and dress himself up in the most fantastic garments. In short, he would dress himself as a young schoolgirl, but under his skirt, instead of panties, he would put a baby's napkin. This he would wet, and then proceed into the lounge, where his lady friend would be dressed as a school-mistress-cum-children's nurse. She would say to him: 'Come over here. Have you wet yourself again?' And he would display all the appropriate gestures of contrition and shame. She would then bend him over her knee, take off the napkin, and smack him. Perhaps it is unnecessary for me to go into further details of these extraordinary proceedings, which occupied the whole of an afternoon and evening. Of course, this man was repeating some fantastic experiences and traumas of his early life, rather muddled up together. I am here tempted to comment that the popular horror of sexual abnormalities, which is so widespread among relatively normal people, is to my mind a revelation on their part, on the part of the so-called normal public, of similar infantile fixations, but in their case repressed. In short, those who exhibit undue horror at the peculiarities of harmless sexual performances can be regarded as themselves also very young indeed. Such feelings of horror extending to every form of sexuality are more usual among neurotics than are perversions; sometimes we have both in the same person. Indeed, neurosis has been said to be the negation of perversion. The psychopathology of both neurosis and perversion has the same basis in trends that are normal in the young and are called psychosexual 'component instincts'. These are developmentally earlier than mature adult genital sexuality, and if unduly emphasised, fixated and left by the wayside, can reveal their accumulated tensions either positively (expression) in the form of peculiar, incomplete or perverted, sexual behaviour, or negatively (repression) in the form of undue horror and anxiety, or simply as anxiety without any idea of what the anxiety is about.

Amongst the earliest of the protective defences of the mind against anxiety is the mechanism of splitting, or dissociating painful and unpleasant emotional reactions and the phantasies connected with them from the rest of the personality. The defence of splitting, according to some psychoanalysts the earliest defensive mechanism, can reach such a degree that it would seem that almost the whole of the individual's emotional life is split off from his reality contacts. If the ego shares in this splitting process, we have a condition analogous to that which is said by some psychoanalysts to prevail in earliest babyhood. It is regarded as a reaction back to the most primitive self-protective state. The sufferer may be unable to deal normally with the realities of life, indeed he may withdraw from practically all reality contacts. This is a mental condition known as schizophrenia and, in its clinically recognisable form, such persons are not ordinarily part of the analyst's clientele. Nevertheless, it may be said that none of us is entirely free from some minor element of this process. Indeed, to my mind, introversion is a slight, if in a limited degree useful and beneficial, minor movement of this nature, and the introverted person is commonly a better analytical subject than the extreme extrovert. Any tendency to schizoid ego-splitting or to hysteria-induced multiple personality, which a patient may possess, is reduced in the course of analytical treatment, which is likely to synthesise the various dissociated parts of his personality into a more united whole. Persons tend to become 'more and more themselves' in spite of exhibiting a series of obsessional defences against being themselves, and in spite of obsessional elements entering, often unwelcome, into what should be a united picture.

Psychopathic personalities, delusional systems and minor psychoses in general are very resistant to psychotherapeutic amelioration. Curious as it may sound, my experience as an analyst has taught me that the one thing people are most keen about is sticking to their particular psychosis. There is a tacit recognition of this in political, social or colonial life. When we rule a primitive race, we usually tell our agents and administrators not on any account to try to influence the people's religion, or to interfere with their religious rites and customs, however crazy they are. It seems that why people are so keen about sticking to their psychoses is because this enables them to live emotionally, and that is gratifying, rather than to live rationally, which is not so gratifying. A patient. who was particularly difficult in a social sense told me at a very late stage of his analysis: 'If you stir people up emotionally when they are very young, like I was stirred up by all the disturbances in my childhood, *all* they need is emotional relief, that's what you're telling me I can't have.' The sort of emotional relief this patient was keen about was expressing his aggressive hate all over the place, with the result that people were afraid of him. He continued: 'It's a sort of brain-washing you are giving me. And how *cruel* it is you'll never know.' He added fervently: 'I hope to God you'll never know.' In other words, sanity is a very 'cruel' thing to inflict upon those who deviate from it, even if the degree of deviation is slight, great, or merely normal. Only analysis can teach us the truth of these revolutionary conclusions.

To avoid any misconception, I must reaffirm that the majority of the patients coming to an analyst belong to the category or categories which I first mentioned in this list, namely those of internal tensions without symptoms or internal tensions with symptoms of anxiety, or with symptoms fairly near to their anxiety origins, such as those of hysteria. One gets a certain number of cases of hysteria in married women, which appear to be due, very largely at least, to the relative impotence of their husbands, although of course they may have in most cases some psychopathic trend which this unsatisfactoriness of the husband has brought out. Nevertheless, it is a real factor in the causation of a certain number of cases of hysteria. It is extraordinary the number of women married for quite long periods whom we discover still to be virgins—even after sixteen years of marriage. But the most extraordinary thing about these cases is that very often they have no conception of the facts. Some of them have even imagined that their husband's fumbling was what was meant by coitus. The variety of symptomatic manifestations that certain cases can portray is of course limitless. The tragedy of it is that it is often impossible to treat the husband, for his method of 'dealing' with his trouble has often been that of hoodwinking himself and everybody else regarding the unsatisfactory nature of his psychosexual constitution. Impotence can vary from absolute impotence to every degree of imperfection in psychosexual activity, and it is remarkable how it can go unrecognised by both parties.

Different doctors use a variety of methods in the treatment of psychologically disturbed or ill patients. There is a large group which confines its activities to drugs and physical methods, but strictly speaking these are acting more as physicians than as psychotherapists. Different psychotherapists have differences in their methods of treating psychoneurotic patients. There are a few who still use hypnosis, suggestion, reassurance and so on. Most psychotherapists now regard these early methods as superficial, unsatisfactory and out of date, and rely chiefly if not exclusively on a technique of analysis. That is to say, a technique designed to trace the *unconscious* source of the trouble, and to reveal the mechanisms whereby it came into existence, thus increasing the patient's insight, and as it were enabling his own ego to deal with the trouble within his own psyche.

The technique amounts largely to letting the patient be himself and encouraging him if necessary to express himself verbally during his sessions with the analyst. The difficulty is often that the patient is himself in the habit of reinforcing a lot of defensive processes, as though he were chiefly concerned to resist his own naturalness. Therefore, although the analyst attempts first and foremost to be an impassive spectator, as it were, and although he may find little difficulty in the anamnesis, that is to say, in taking a detailed history of the origin of the illness, going back as far as the patient's conscious memory will permit, this always proves in due course to be not enough. Sooner or later the analyst finds that he has to deal with involuntary resistance on the part of the patient's psyche. In an endeavour to expose, analyse and get through this resistance the means the analyst uses can be summarised in the terms 'relaxation and free association of thought'. The latter is commonly called the basic rule of analysis.

It is extraordinary that in spite of all the will in the world to co-operate, involuntary resistance keeps interfering with the analytical process. This phenomenon too can commonly be regarded as a reaction to anxiety. Even after months of treatment, when she thought she was co-operating to the limits of her ability, a patient told me 'but doctor, if I relaxed and gave in to my feelings, I would be a semi-invalid,' indicating that she was maintaining a state of apparent health by dint of continuous stress and strain. Excessive stress and strain cannot be maintained without penalties such as visceroptosis, (from which she was suffering), and in any case it cannot be maintained all the time. Therefore this patient periodically relapses into a temporary phase of invalidism, accompanied by abdominal pain.

One of the objects of analysis is to discover the source from which a patient's anxiety springs. In due course, with the removal of resistances and increasing freedom of relaxation and association of thought, one learns not only the content of consciousness but also the content of the unconscious phantasies responsible for the Anxiety State and its symptoms. Such insight puts the ego in a better position to deal appropriately with the needs of the natural instincts and impulses, and to adapt the environment to them or to adapt them to the environment, instead of trying ineffectively to maintain unnecessary barriers.

I think of a particular patient whose analysis revealed that throughout life, even from childhood, his sensible endeavour has been to take precautions against his instincts coming out and expressing themselves. This struggle seems to have reached its zenith at puberty in connection with his impulse to masturbate, and subsequently in connection with his impulse towards sexual relationship with the opposite sex. It is difficult to describe how the whole of his life has been an emphasis on precautionary measures to keep his libido from driving him into implementing any such tendencies. Analysis reveals that all this is connected with his unconscious phantasy. The ingredients of this phantasy can be traced back to the Oedipus level of development, where the nuclear content of his unconscious is shown to consist of incestuous drives, omnipotent and therefore murderous—and consequent castration anxiety.

To avoid this terror in the unconscious, he has instituted what might be called a life-long process of self-castration, coupled with an extraordinary degree of anxiety. He has tried to placate his life urges by various displaced forms of activity, much in the way that all normal people do—but, on the eve of, for example, a holiday abroad, the morbid nature of his unconscious reveals itself in an outcrop of excessive anxiety symptoms threatening to prevent his departure, Analysis revealed that the distant country he was flying to symbolised his mother, and the pleasure he would get on holiday symbolised the incestuous act. He was nearly rendered impotent in the anticipation of this excitement.

His dreams reveal a succession of such tendencies, sometimes displaced on to asexual symbols, but sometimes frankly sexual, in which the striving for pleasure quickly gives place to the most acute anxiety imaginable, coupled with what could only be called 'castration symbolism'. The boat he was travelling on rots away and breaks into pieces; the aeroplane he was flying in gets loose at all the joints, crashes, and he is burnt alive. Nevertheless, he has struggled on with this unsatisfactory life, trying to get what pleasure he can and being periodically overtaken by this acute anxiety emanating from his unconscious castration complex. Such a psychic structure can only have its origin in the very early organisation of the psyche at what is called the Oedipus level. In the course of his analysis, this structure is seen to extend back right down to his infancy, but a full revelation of such things is not possible until the patient has reached a complete transference stage of analysis and begun actually to feel the hopes and fears, loves and hates, in connection with the figure of his own analyst. The danger is of such cases (when their anxiety is lessened and their repressed libido liberated) breaking out prematurely into inappropriate extra-analytical activities. However, even this in some cases is preferable to life-long mental *and physical* invalidism. And after all it is not so different from what all one's normal unanalysed brothers and sisters are doing all the time!

As recollection proceeds to deeper and earlier levels of development, the analyst is unwittingly placed in the role of the first objects in the patient's life, namely the parent or parents of his infancy. When the analyst is in a position to expose and interpret the pattern of this psychological projection, analysis has gone a long way towards bringing first causes into the patient's conscious mind and creating the opportunity for readjustment more in keeping with the patient's adult ego and reason.

A certain amount of benefit is almost inevitable in most cases. In my opinion, degrees of failure are often attributable to the fact that not every emotional reactive pattern is the product of causes within the infant's lifetime, even if we go back as far as breast feeding. Last month the father of a child of six years told me that she is now exhibiting a phobia of dogs which *he* displayed at her age. This is the child's sixth neurotic symptom identical with a series which he displayed in his infancy. The conclusion seems to me inescapable: that like the instincts, some of these reactive patterns had been created in past generations, and at least the tendency towards them inherited by the unfortunate patient as a predisposition to neurosis.

Nevertheless, analysis appears to provide the greatest hope so far of readjustment and amelioration in the profoundest sense. It often proves that there is not all that difference between, for instance, hysteria and the emotional drives which are the essential dynamic value of life itself. It can even be argued with some justification that you must have hysteria, or something very like it, to achieve anything emotional in this life, or indeed perhaps to achieve anything at all.

CHAPTER XVII

THE PSYCHOLOGY OF LOVE

THE late Dr. Groddeck tells us that the first lesson for every doctor to learn is that *he* cannot cure anybody of anything. As mentioned, Dr. Groddeck is the originator of the concept that we are 'lived by the It' (or id). It is from him that I borrowed the title of this book, parodying its scientific value with the phrase 'My Life', in order to leave no doubt that my intention was autobiographical.

Having told us that we cannot cure anybody of anything, Dr. Groddeck implies that we can only utilise Nature's forces. The psychiatrist should know this better than any other doctor. He knows his limitations and is perhaps the most careful of all doctors never to accept the role of 'wise man', which some patients would thrust upon him. Nevertheless, if one spends one's days in listening to the free association of thought of a succession of persons, abnormal and approximately normal, one finds oneself acquiring an insight into the forces and mechanisms which move them. More than this, one finds oneself acquiring an insight, directly and indirectly, into the forces and mechanisms which move every human being. Eventually, through this, one acquires an insight into the very origin and nature of the structure of civilisation, its development through the ages, savage rites, anthropological customs, ancient and modern history, the origin of all human biases and beliefs, and through these, into the very fabric of our everyday life together with that of our cultural organisations and institutions. One reaches the stage when one cannot even read the leader in a newspaper without automatically distinguishing cold fact from emotional admixture, without seeing something objective and something subjective, without discerning defensive mechanisms as well as emotional outlets.

After all, every patient arrives full of inhibitions and defences, and the technique of analysis is to analyse defensive processes, remove unnecessary resistances, enable the mind to be conscious of what is in it, and so, where advantageous and advisable, to free the expression of emotions and feelings more and more.

Forces and mechanisms are revealed, which would otherwise be unrecognised or slow in coming to light, or confused; deeper levels of defence are revealed and previously concealed forces emerge. All these are soon discovered to be common to every individual and to the movements of the mind, single and corporate. It is indeed a fascinating study, especially when it is found to have unlimited application to all things human.

When I was about to take up analysis as a profession, a doctor friend of the family asked my sister what her brother was proposing to specialise in, and when she told him, he got terribly excited and said to her: 'For heaven's sake, don't let him do it. He will be lost to everybody. You will practically never see him again!' Of course, this was an exaggeration, but there is something in the point of view. It may be asked, how can one be expected to get excited about ordinary amateurish psychological interests when one is professionally engaged in the deeper levels of the mind from which everything springs. I am here suggesting in parenthesis that most of our social conversations and personal interest in one another are psychological interests of a relatively superficial nature, contaminated by our own unresolved biases and limited by our defensive mechanisms.

During the course of analysis one sees these in an unmistakably vivid light. One sees not only how the prevailing mood of a patient has been influenced, if not determined by his early upbringing, but also how his way of looking at things, his very character, has been formed—largely out of defensive processes. For example, only today, when I pointed out (quite unemotionally, of course) to a patient that throughout the session he had been trying to provoke a row with me, he gained a little insight and said: 'If I had taken all father gave me, if I had allowed all his criticisms and remarks to pass unanswered, I would have been a *depressive* all my days.' This patient is certainly not a depressive but even this little remark of his may suggest to us how a depressed person can be created. He went on to say: 'My aggressive reaction to father was necessary for survival. As you see, I have survived—but with no place in the world.' This patient's home life seems to have been an almost continuous ROW between different members of the family—mother and father at the head. Towards the conclusion of the session, I said: 'You have very much the same disposition and temperament as your father. You are handing to people in your vicinity what he handed to you. Perhaps if they take it lying down, *they* become depressive! If they react defensively, as you reacted to your father, then there is a row. That is how and why you have rows with people wherever you go. It is their only alternative to becoming depressive. You either make a person into a depressive or you create a row—that is why you have, as you say "no place in the world".'

This patient retorted: 'You are asking me to retain what is within me, and which I *cannot retain*. If I retained the tension, I would become a depressive. You are asking me to become a depressive.'

This is not a very good example of analysis as it belongs essentially to a terminal stage of ego-modification. I think there are grounds for doubting whether any such technique should be attempted, unless we want the patient to conclude his treatment. However, it is probably easier to understand because it resembles ordinary naïve attempts to modify a person. Intrapsychic conflict is revealed in infinite variety throughout the daily sessions of analysis, until it is borne home upon the analyst that all these emotional actions and reactions are the very fabric out of which the World of Man, its history and culture, its successive customs, peace and war, are built.

The analyst's business is to study his patient and to understand this interplay of emotional forces without himself partaking emotionally of them, or at least without giving any sign that they tend to cause emotional reactions in himself. If he has an emotional life at all during his work, it is only as it were by proxy, and must remain unexpressed, unrelieved. Otherwise he will be entering the 'dog-fight' himself, instead of remaining in his proper role as a scientific observer and interpreter of it. He will have lost his position as a scientist or analyst and become instead merely a liver, one of the dogs.

Well, now, the truth I want to come to in this chapter is this: fundamentally the analyst *is* one of the dogs. Fundamentally of course he is a human being like every other human being, like every analysand, and as such he needs an adequate amount of emotional outlet upon the same level. He was biologically created and

P

developed in exactly the same way as everybody else. Whatever his scientific study, intellectual or emotional *interest*, he must remain like all other organisms basically immersed in the emotional reliefs that come through living and the processes of life.

Ever and anon during analysis, one patient after another comes to the realisation that the cultural, scientific and other interests which he has adopted from his mentors, or which have been forced upon him, are really only substitutes or pretences, containing at the most only a modicum of the emotional intensity and instinctual drive which remains massively at the biological level. The process starts when the infant exchanges direct emotional gratification, such as breast-feeding, with a psuedo-gratification with some substitutive object, such as a toy. Subsequently culture grows upon him with a vast succession of toys and substitutive interests, building up all the gadgets and paraphernalia of civilisation. He will only pretend to be content with these. Deep down, the fundamental urges are still building up tensions and beating against the barriers. They will find an outlet sooner or later, otherwise we would not be here to tell the tale. The primitive forces of life are not permanently diverted by the substitutive make-believes or 'fob-offs'.

Analysis of patients reveals that my epitomised examples here given are over-simplified, and it is not so simple a matter as *instinct* gratification or *instinct* repression. On account of early frustrations, complicated reactive patterns have developed incredibly early in life, and there is a strong tendency in every individual to act out his own particular reactive patterns. I have come to regard these as the first fruits of frustrations, differing from the instincts in two particulars only. One is that they are not necessarily exhibited in that (instinct) *form*, and two, that their elaborate construction is peculiar to the particular individual. The compulsions and obsessions they lead to can be very complicated and impossible to unravel without the application of analytical technique and insight. Even activities which have the stamp of the most fundamental biological or instinctual urges may not be what they seem. They may themselves be uncomfortable substitutions for the acquired reactive pattern of that particular individual.

For instance, a patient, a married man, tells me that his sexual relationship with his wife, although he is apparently potent and successful, is all a make-believe, and fails to bring him real psychosexual satisfaction. In this connection he says to me: 'The reason I am ill, doctor, is because *all* my activities are substitutions. Substitutions for true, ordinary human relationship. In my life there is no sexual fulfilment and no emotional stability. From the time my mother frustrated me (by loving my brother more than me) everything has been a substitute as far as I can remember. The result today is that my wife (although she does not know it) is not enjoyed. She is there only as a foil. The prevailing feeling of my life is the feeling of perpetual and intolerable frustration.'

This man's illness will be found on further analysis to spring from the frustration of his earliest infantile phantasies in connection with his mother. He could not get the degree of love and freedom which he required and he could not tolerate the frustration without repercussions amounting to illness.

We appear to accept that which is sold us, or rather that which is thrust upon us, and to make it our own, but something deep down feels that the whole thing is a substitution for what we really want. We embrace civilisation and culture and pretend to ourselves and to others that they are better than life, but the truth appears to be that we only do these things in so far as 'life' is denied us, in so far as we are frustrated from achieving our original emotional omnipotence. Our Oedipus fulfilment is frustrated and henceforth we are making the best of an indifferent world, or pretending to do so.

Analysis may suggest to us that the elaborate edifice of civilisation is built upon a very flimsy defensive foundation. Perhaps it would be better to regard it as a garment in which we dress ourselves, an appearance rather than a reality. Nevertheless, it is a structure which reveals a good deal of the nature of the hidden animal which lies underneath it, the denial of which has gone into its making.

To put it shortly, investigating and studying the processes of mental life is not in itself essentially an emotional experience. It is, or should be, a scientific process, although probably some modicum of emotional experience is impossible to exclude from any of our cultural interests. In some respects this cultural interest, like any other scientific study, and like all intellectual and civilised preoccupations, is essentially a substitution. It does not prove to be an adequate substitution for life itself.

In these pages, I have tried to give a slight indication of the daily occupation and interests of my life as a psychiatrist and analyst, if only to compare and contrast them with my early years as a general practitioner, but I am not going to pretend that these interests comprised or comprise the whole of my life, and as this book is essentially an autobiography, I must here admit that the ordinary things of life were certainly not excluded. In the process of following my professional interests, I had to be protected from the intrusions and interruptions of the world around me: telephone, door bells, and a hundred and one other frustrations and interruptions, not to speak of the complicated structure of a professional business: appointments, letters, correspondence, accounts, bills and the innumerable ordinary things of life.

More than a decade had passed since the birth of my daughter, and the young woman whom friends had introduced to me, and installed as my secretary, had succeeded in making herself the inconspicuous but essential protector of my professional welfare. Like many men in such a position, I was slow to appreciate how excellent were her services, and how indispensable were not only the work she did, but her very presence in the establishment.

Inevitable vacations from work, such as were occasioned by Christmas, summer and public holidays, I regarded merely as opportunities for some literary work, and here too my invaluable secretary was the obvious answer to every problem.

Having no important attachments in life except my now elderly mother, who was living at my married sister's house in the country, and my two children, now developing in boarding schools, and a few friends that one had time to meet only occasionally, my secretary and I were thrown more and more together. It became quite apparent that her main, if not exclusive interest in life, was her work, and my work, and enabling me to keep at it in spite of the difficulties of the latter years of the war. It was only many years later, in looking back upon things, that I came to realise how unconcerned both she and I had been in enduring the menace of flying bombs and V.2's in the heart of London, for the sake of keeping up the work. We were both so fully occupied that the thought of leaving what we regarded as the main business of our lives never so much as occurred to us.

All I can say about my second marriage is that in contra-distinction to my first, it appeared to have no starting point whatsoever. There was certainly no sudden falling in love at first sight, and no sudden falling in love at all. It seemed to occur simply and gradually, out of service and propinquity. I do not think either of us knew when or how it came about. It must have been simply that as the weeks, months and years of our relationship grew, so we gradually and imperceptibly grew closer and closer together. Maybe the conscious mind was fixed upon the things that are Caesar's, while, all unseen and all unbeknown to us, our unconscious natures were moving us closer together. Perhaps when I was younger, I was unconsciously seeking a glamourous dynamic extrovert; but in later years I tended to be drawn to the less superficial qualities of the calm, quiet, unselfish, but no less delightful helpmeet. Biological forces go on, and have their way, whether or not the conscious levels of the mind are otherwise engaged. Indeed, the essential thesis of this chapter is that while our conscious minds are preoccupied with substitutions, the fundamental forces that are the real life, the true life, continue to operate as they have done for the past four hundred million years, since the coelacanthus and before. Indeed, it would prove impossible to put on this camouflage dress called civilisation if there were not a body (i.e. an animal) on which to put it.

One of the many differences between my second marriage and my first was that, far from it being an exciting distraction from my analytical and professional work, it was, on the contrary, the very opposite, namely a facilitation of my every scientific interest and endeavour. My first marriage in my youth, however delightful, made everything almost intolerably difficult for me, whereas my second marriage in my middle age smoothed the path of life, material, physical and mental, to a degree that at first seemed incredible.

Nevertheless, the reality story is not yet fully told. I do not suppose I am the only man of the middle fifties who has married a woman twenty-five years his junior, imagining that she had no desire or ambition different from his own, only to discover in due course that she had at least one ambition which he had not thought of, an ambition common to almost all newly married young women. In due course it transpired that she did not think a childless marriage was a complete marriage, and as she had throughout served my every wish, I could hardly deny her the only wish which was truly her own. Again the years, and even the months, proved that she was more right than I could ever have imagined, for the infant, now a little girl of seven years, has become more important not only to her, but to me also, than anything else in our lives. Indeed, so right did my wife prove to be in this respect, that I could hardly doubt the rightness of her subsequent desire to add yet another to this family! In fact, there could hardly be a doubt that one child being a source of so much happiness, another would do less than add to it.

And so it is that the plans one makes and the interests one pursues on a conscious level, professional, scientific and research interests, are revealed in the long run as substitutes for something more fundamental, something which the young woman may realise more acutely than the middle-aged man. Man proposes; woman disposes! Man, or at any rate professional man, has proceeded so far along the path of substitutive values . . . but fortunately not too far to be called back in some respects to the true values of life itself.

There is indeed no substitute for living. Not even science. My experience has been that science can be added to living only if living has itself been adequately and satisfactorily provided for. Science is possible only when the fundamental needs of life are sufficiently secure to obviate undue anxiety; only when one is tolerably healthy and happy. Here too, my experience has been that my original theme was correct when I emphasised that life is not life without growth and reproduction. Life is never standing still. It has either to be expanding and growing or else it is contracting, and dying out.

The psychoanalytical theory that love is a sort of combination of the mutually exclusive processes of 'object relationship' and 'identification', seems to me little more than an attempt to bring it into line with psychoanalytical concepts. To my mind, this is an inadequate and misleading presentation of the fundamental, unconscious nature of love. Though I can welcome the statement that 'one can speak of love only when consideration of the object goes so far that one's own satisfaction is impossible without satisfying the object too' (Fenichel, P. 84), I feel that this states an attribute of a highly integrated process, a sort of end-product, and tells us little of the anatomy of love, of its basic structure, its origins or fundamental nature.

The primary levels of love, the essential nature of the process, begin with unconscious mental mechanisms of an automatic and primitive kind. Admittedly 'identification' enters into the process, and also admittedly one naturally 'loves' an 'object' that gratifies. It is indeed from these basic mechanisms that unconscious association of thought leads to *fetishistic* developments of great variety and complexity. The mother's nipple (and from association, the mother), or other early gratifying object, turns up in a limitless number of disguises throughout the individual's life.

The enormous amount of fetishistic influence in falling in love, and indeed in any sexual attraction and stimulation, has not been adequately admitted or recognised consciously—though almost everything in our civilisation, from the manufacture of cosmetics to the shops in Regent Street and Mayfair (conspicuously dress and jewellery), bears witness to its *unconscious* 'recognition'. I am using the concept of fetishism in a very loose way, and I shall now ask the reader to learn what I mean by the term, as I cannot otherwise explain the psychology of love.

Fetishism is defined by Freud as a substitution for the normal sexual object, a substitution which is totally unfit for the normal sexual aim. I am sure that precise definitions, though very useful for theoretical, and perhaps for scientific, purposes in some circumstances, have enormous disadvantages which I believe have seldom been properly or fully expounded. They are like the codification of the law; one grows to think that the definition is something in nature, and loses sight of the fact that nature never invented the definition. Natural phenomena merge one into another. When we make a definition, we often select and isolate a particular phenomenon, or part of a phenomenon, and encase it in a rigid wall as though it had no connection with the surroundings. In this way, we misrepresent the phenomenon, and produce a misconception of nature as a whole. The precise definitions of the law are a wonderful example of this.

I would like to leave out of my definition of fetishism the matter of the object being totally unfit for the normal sexual aim. I do not quite know what this means, 'unfit for the normal sexual aim'! Of course, we know that the most astonishing examples of fetishism, of pathological states of sexual attraction—often exclusively to some such bizarre object as mackintoshes—are the sort of grounds upon which this definition has been formulated; but what the definition hides from our realisation is that there is *every degree* of this sort of thing, and that it is all these multitudinous, minor degrees and varieties which not only exist in every normal mind, but add up to form, in my opinion, the general quality of sexual attraction in every object '*fit* for the normal sexual aim'.

As with every conscious presentation, there are various levels of interpretation corresponding to the various levels within the mind, and the interpretations are not necessarily mutually exclusive. Various levels of interpretation are possible just in the same way as a screen memory may refer to a certain age and development, and be quite true as far as it goes, while at the same time the complex or emotional drama which it is screening is also true, is in fact the same thing at a deeper level or earlier period of life.

My theory is that the qualities of an object (a person) that cause it (him or her) to be a sexual stimulus, or an object of attraction or of love, are manifold and are all what I would call *fetishistically determined* with or without some basic reality aspect. The fetish has, at one level of interpretation, been defined as some object, quality or attribute originally pertaining to the mother, which became at an early age associated with sexual feelings— sexual feelings which may not in the first instance have been aroused specifically by that object, quality or attribute, but which were in some way connected with it, perhaps by a coincidence in time between the observation of the object and the experience of the feeling. It is thus, in this sense, a conditioned response to the object. Groddeck has said that falling in love is most intimately connected with smell—presumably often unconsciously. We know on the other hand that however much smell figures in strict fetishism—and it does figure very prominently in a lot of fetishistic perversions—it is certainly not the only and usually not even the necessary qualification. There are limitless ingredients in fetishistic attraction, especially in the sense in which I wish to use it, as pertaining to all sexual attraction.

They are, almost certainly, all attributes associated with the mother in infancy or mother surrogates, and I am inclined to say that they include everything that attracts. Cases have been instanced where a person was sexually stimulated by another person's paroxysms of coughing—traced back to the paroxysms of coughing which this individual's mother suffered from, especially during his early life. I am instancing this to show how far the mind can go in borrowing ingredients from the mother to qualify an object as sexually attractive. You have only to add that association can be by contrast as well as by similarity and identity, to realise that every quality in a person that stimulates another sexually, or causes him to be attracted to her or to love her, can be a result of conditioning from the earlier stages of development when mother was the love object.

Now, the point I wish to make is that while one's reason should tell one that certain attributes of an object have a reality value, and others, however stimulating, are relatively valueless, the emotional excitement or disturbance aroused by these various qualities is in no wise necessarily related to their real value. I have known men to marry women because they had a beautiful head of hair or a shapely ankle, a nice leg, prominent breasts, a pretty face or a certain type of face, a way of moving, a musical voice, an indefinable manner, and a million and one comparable attributes, tangible and intangible—why, men have even married women because they used a certain variety of scent!—none of which had anything whatsoever to do with real value. What they had to do with, to my mind, is a mechanism of conditioning comparable to that of fetishism, and closely related to the individual's predilection for part-object love. This may be more credible when we mention breasts; I have written a small book to show how it applies to *hair*, but it applies equally to everything. Psychoanalysis can produce much evidence to suggest that the fetish, or for that matter the part-object, may be a reassuring substitute for the mother's missing phallus, though it would be more credible to those who have a resistance to such interpretations to go to a still deeper level and suggests that it is a substitute for the mother's missed breast or missed nipple.

However, we need not go to any such deep levels of interpretation to explain my theory that love and sexual attraction are based upon a conglomeration of diffuse fetishisms, using the term in my loose general sense, for which I think there is ample justification. I feel that this attitude to the subject has an application to our attenuated and diffuse sexual life throughout all its cultural ramifications. The emphasis on the distinction between the sexes—the clothes a woman wears in their marked divergence from male attire, her hair fashion, her shoes, her stockings, her underwear, her ornaments, everything about her from top to toe—is all an elaborate system, however, unconsciously instigated, of trying to encourage fetishistic attraction. All these artificialities that are perhaps the characteristic of our culture, not excluding scent, powder and cosmetics, are all based upon the festishistic nature of attraction between the sexes. One has only to reflect upon all the establishments whose function it is to serve these proclivities of civilised people, to realise that the ramifications of this unrealistic, but emotionally and sexually important element in our lives, appear to be limitless.

What part has real value to do with sexual attraction or with love? In the light of these considerations, one may be excused for wondering whether it has any influence at all. At least one important consideration has been omitted. We know, for instance, that a person under analysis is liable to acquire a 'transference' towards his or her analyst. In fact, it has often been regretted that the analyst cannot remain, like the Catholic priest at confessional, completely unseen (and perhaps unheard) as it has been suggested that the phenomenon of transference might then be facilitated. Admittedly transference is not wholly positive (love), but sooner or later includes negative elements, or feelings of hatred. Indeed it is these latter, sometimes associated with deprivations ('castrations') on the part of the hated parent-images, which are responsible for pain and illness, in the same way as love, associated with gratifications (starting at the breast) from the loved parent-images, are responsible for pleasure and health. The psychoneurotic patient particularly has regressed emotionally to his early childhood and the feelings he has for his analyst are seen to be nothing more or less than a re-living of his infant-parent relationship. In the light of this revelation love is shown to contain important ingredients of one's emotional attachments to parents going right back to the insecurities and dependencies of infancy and babyhood. Therefore, one might argue that love, like hate, is something independent of appearances and their fetishistics implications, that the transference, no less than the fetishistic or part-object influence, is independent of any reality-based objective assessment of the object or person valued. The necessary qualification is that he should not have interfered with or prevented the unfolding of this infant-parent-based tendency in the other. In short, the loving of a person would appear to be more a subjective than an objective matter. It is the quality of loving, of the need to love, within the subject rather than any lovable attribute of the object, which are the matters of prime importance. If a person has a need, an emotional need, to love, he will attach it to some object (i.e. person or dog) without necessarily having discovered or assessed any objective, reason-based valuation.

Thus we may conclude that in so far as the phenomenon of love is fetishistically determined (and I am suggesting that this is the usual basis of it), it has in common with the phenomenon of transference ('loving' an unknown and perhaps unseen person— c.f. God) the fact that both are subjectively conditioned, and both are completely irrational as regards objective valuation. We may conclude also that fetishism, love and transference have a common basis in the revival of early patterns, originally connected with the parent or with some part or attribute of the parent.

One can go further than this and suggest that the *absence* of the fetish (or fetishes), be it lipstick or hair, can be reacted to as to a defect or deformity, a castration symbol, and arouse castration-anxiety, thus spoiling the attraction and causing bad feelings to displace good ones. There is abundant clinical evidence of this phenomenon. I have a patient, for instance, who is not sexually interested in his wife, or in any woman, *unless she is wearing a mackintosh*. In his case she has to be wearing lipstick as well, and then his excitement knows no bounds! Do not laugh too heartily until you have told me how you would react to a lady who was totally bald.

The search for *beauty* is nothing more or less than an attempt to avoid castration symbols and consequent castration anxiety. I have a patient who in his dreams, as in his real life, is repeatedly discovering some blemish (ugliness, deformity, thinness, or even a mole) in his lady love, with an immediate cessation of all his sexual interest in her. (Psychosexual impotence in men is commonly precipitated by the women's absence of penis.) He is like Don Juan, for ever searching for the 'perfect' woman. It seems that he is looking for the mother-image of his infancy before he discovered that she was without a phallus (i.e. 'castrated'). Curiously enough, while beauty implies the absence of castration symbolism, that is to say no terrifying blemish or castration, it does not necessarily seem to suggest the presence of a phallus. The presence of a phallus can suggest father's castrating phallus, and be as off-putting as the blemish. Take off my beautiful lady's nose and she is spoiled, but give her an enormously large one and she is equally spoiled. Grotesque figures in a dream always symbolise genitals and may combine phallic and castration symbolism. They are often more displeasing than pleasing. When Keats wrote his famous lines:

' "Beauty is truth, truth beauty",—that is all
Ye know on earth, and all ye need to know.'

he was endeavouring to reassure himself that the *absence of castration was the truth*, i.e. that there is no such thing as castration—(by 'castration' one means also: annihilation, bad things or bad happenings)—and therefore that there was no need for (castration-)anxiety. A reassurance of this nature is necessary before we can feel the security essential for pleasure and enjoyment; that is why we 'need to know' it, and why it is 'all we need to know'.

We are talking about automatic reactions and operations due chiefly to mental mechanisms which are not necessarily conscious or reasonable. Nevertheless, they are mental mechanisms, and, like instincts, they have connections with the past, connections which may be intimately associated with conditions for survival. Is it reasonable to prefer salmon to cod, or to prefer meat to fish, or spinach to turnips, or any of these things to the equivalent nourishment in the form of a tablet? Well, we don't bother to answer. All we know is that one or other of these gives us pleasure and another does not, or may even give us disgust. According to our pleasure, we will react favourably, not only pyschologically but even physiologically. Generally speaking, we will not only enjoy but also digest the food we like, but to any food, however nutritious, to which we react with disgust, however unreasonably, our stomach may do the same, and vomiting instead of benefit result.

Thus, our emotional life, whether it has to do with eating, with sexuality or with love, is based upon reactions belonging to a deeper level than those of our reasoning faculties, very often, no doubt, sounder than those of our reasoning faculties. After all, reason is only a late development, whereas these other mechanisms have seen us through the ages. It is thanks to them that we have survived, therefore we should be very sure before we trust a new friend, such as reason, in preference to the old ones.

It would seem that our difficulties in all our adjustments in life may be regarded as due to a conflict between these rival claims to priority, the old and the new. We are only too apt to think that it is reason that determines our actions, or determines those that matter, but let us ask, remembering Samuel Butler, what determines the pumping action of our heart. This may remind us that all the fundamental activities and behaviours within us (and, I would add, without) are pre-determined by instincts and by conditioned reactions which have priority to reason. Reason, more particularly in the light of analytical revelation, is very rarely trustworthy. Most commonly, it is itself conditioned by our emotional biases and needs, a tool or servant in the hands of forces far older and far stronger than itself.

Thus, for me all this life of ours, with its various activities, habits, conventions, institutions and beliefs, was a subject of research in the light of analytical insight. It was a phenomenon of nature, like the growth of a plant, to be studied scientifically, and the laws by which it reacted observed and understood, just as one would observe and understand any other group of natural phenomena. With a sufficient knowledge of the basis and source of things, the ills of humanity, emotional, mental and organic, would be as fully explained and understood as normality and health. In fact, there was plenty within one's researches to suggest that abnormalities were easier to understand; they showed up the mechanisms more clearly than did normality, but there was not a lot between them. They were all parts of the same complicated machine, just as determined as the phenomena in any other department of nature, just as subject to the law of cause and effect as were the phenomena of physics and chemistry.

Thus it came about that while I was being analysed and obtaining insight into a world of nature within myself, which had hitherto been practically unsuspected, while I was applying a similar technique to my patients at the Tavistock Clinic and elsewhere, I was daily accumulating more and more material for my research and understanding of the riddle of nature. All science is one, and the fact that I had chosen one of the most intangible and difficult sub-divisions of the field of enquiry, namely that of psychology, for the purpose of my investigations, may have had advantages as well as disadvantages. I had often thought, and still think, that I should have stuck to physics, which I first encountered on entering St. Thomas's Medical School, and of which I discovered immediately that I had a facile understanding. Maybe this psychological study was too extraordinarily difficult. One's own emotions were so apt to get mixed up with it. In physics, one would have had the advantage of dealing with inanimate matter, and no excuse for emotional entanglements! But perhaps this very difficulty, inherent in the subject of psychology, made it not only particularly intriguing, but also more promising. It certainly appeared to be a less explored field, less successfully explored because the investigator had inevitably become tangled up with his own emotions, and too blinded by them to see the scientific truth. In all other studies, the investigator had put aside his emotional life, to escape from emotion, a sort of defence against the problems and conflicts within himself; a defence by flight. But here, I found that I had chosen as the object of my scientific research the very source of interference with scientific thought, the tangle of emotions themselves, my tangle of emotions. One of the advantages of this choice was also its main disadvantage. It was related to the question: was it possible to study emotion emotionlessly? Perhaps it is not possible to study anything emotionlessly. The best we can do is the same as everyone else endeavours to do in all departments of life and thought: to try to distinguish between emotional valuations and reason or reality valuations. Science, in contra-distinction to beliefs and legends, emerges only in so far as man is successful in making this distinction. The degree of success is always limited.

In the light of psychology, particularly in the light of analysis, one could see the whole human race, including oneself, driven by forces in which reason was hardly discernible. The behaviour of man, his habits, his customs, his conventions, his institutions, and even, or perhaps particularly, his thoughts and beliefs, were in the mass so obviously a product of inherited and conditioned emotional forces, in the drive and activity of which, any reason which he might possess was swept headlong away, or at the most perverted by them and harnessed to their purpose. All this could be exposed scientifically, accurately. Freud had done an enormous quantity of this, but I soon felt that I did not need to take my data and their scientific assessment from Freud or from any other authority. I meant to find it myself by dint of my own analysis, and by application of the technique to others. Even if I never succeeded in travelling as far as Freud had already travelled, at least it would be my own journey. My mind was so constituted that I could only believe what I discovered and saw for myself.

Thus, in some respects at least they might differ from those of others; they would differ more especially in so far as those of others had been subjectively determined. I felt an enormous need for a science which would explain the activities and beliefs of man, the world of man, in the same way as physics and chemistry explained the behaviour of inanimate nature. I was convinced that such a science was not only possible, but within sight of being expounded exactly, to an advanced degree, to a degree more advanced, more complete, than had ever been done by Freud or by anybody else. Part of my thrill was the idea, which I recognised as comparable to my schoolboy megalomania, that I might be able to go some little way towards doing this. I felt that my predecessors had been too timid, too frightened, perhaps insufficiently convinced to make so bold as to attempt to revolutionise human thought, and to initiate a really far-reaching new orientation for mankind. Freud was the real important pioneer in this enormous field. He had made a great start, but why was his science not developing to elucidate every nook and cranny of human activity and of human thought? I soon began to make notes for the future *magnum opus.* Almost everything that I encountered from the unconscious levels of the mind, my own and other people's, seemed to have its application not only to a better understanding of neurosis, character formation and normality, but also to the unsolved problems of human life and sociology. I was enthralled with my new-found field of research, and at the same time with the progress of my own personal analysis.

I should mention here that not only my inner world appeared to be undergoing changes, developing, emerging to a conscious level, but also the world of my immediate environment, my domestic world, the world of my family and my relationship to it, appeared to become more closely an integral part of me. I felt more complete, more normal by virtue of this state of marriage, my delightful wife and the growing family around us.

This wonderful person we find, suddenly or slowly, and the thought of mating with whom causes our breath to stop and our pulses to bound or to cease, this sudden discovery, this advent of the miracle that promises the end of our exile, the union with another that means life and creates life . . . what is it psychologically, subjectively? Freud has told us. Subjectively it is the re-discovery of the mother whom we lost in infancy, whom we lost with the dissolution or repression of our Oedipus wishes. My need for this reunion may well have been made less urgent and less absolute by virtue of the fact that, apart from sexuality, I had never really lost my original beloved. My mother had always remained an integral part of my life; and my romance, unconscious romance at least, was the unconscious phantasy of journeying with her for ever, through eternity. After all, it would seem that we had come from eternity together, we were eternally (that is throughout my life) together, and would of course face eternity together . . . for evermore. Why should successors or substitutes hold absolute sway when the original, the genuine article, the mother who loved me more than her own soul, was available and actually present.

No matter how private and silent my researches had been, I somehow felt that they would emerge when they had developed sufficiently to rise above the ground; but gradually something else had come about, I had a personal basis or foundation in life, in addition to the pursuit of these intellectual enquiries. I had, as it were, a physical, emotional, instinctual, real basis, I had a body as well as a mind. The love drive, that had caught me up, was an answer, at least on one plane, to a need which I had been trying to ignore, to put aside. Something inside me, everything, was now more comfortable and solid with a firm reality foundation.

I had never endured long periods of emotional wanderings in mid-air, as it were, such as I have seen many poor bachelors and spinsters enduring. I had always felt they were lost souls, exiles. Apart, perhaps, from a taste of it in adolescence, I had never had to put up with the emotional starvation, I almost said agony, of such a state. There had always been my beloved, or more conspicuously, my beloving mother to spoil me, to see that I had every comfort of home, even when I felt I did not want it. Thus, I was never emotionally wandering, there was always that harbour, that resting-place. Had it not been for that, I realise now very clearly indeed that all those years with my mother, though they had provided me with this lair, this really comfortable home life, had at the same time precluded the sexual accompaniments of love, without which such a situation is, physiologically at least, a little unhealthy or injurious.

These disadvantages no longer held good. Now that I had adjusted myself to being mated, I had grown, as it were, into two, I was mated and I was growing, we had grown a family, just as every living thing on this earth, vegetable or animal, is designed by natural laws to grow. Anything, any situation, however seem-ingly agreeable, however consciously agreeable, that prevents this natural biological growth, is comparable to something putting the infant in an iron jacket to prevent the growth and expansion of his body. I say this because I am sure that biologically, and therefore in some sense, however hidden, psychologically, there is no essential dividing line in the biological phenomenon of growth *of* the individual from the egg, and growth *by* the individual, the extension of himself. All life is psychologically, physiologically, chemically, and physically engaged in the fundamental process of growth, of accumulating and ingesting portions of its environment (food) and forming them into more and more of its substance. Reproduction is an inherent part of this process; every cell, whether in multicellular organisms or in a unicellular organism, is multi-plying itself. The advent, in the course of evolution, of specialised organs or a specialised method of reproduction through seed or

Q

egg, is no interruption of the general and fundamental biological process of growth, the most characteristic attribute of all living matter. Therefore, I say that if reproduction is frustrated, whether in human or in bird, psychologically speaking at least, something comparable to an unnatural stoppage of growth is taking place. Psychological repercussions of this, however imperceptible or unconscious, are inevitable.

With my development, perhaps initiated by analysis, but now analytical, biological and natural, I am pleased to be able to say that the old bugbear of my life, the neuralgic attacks, disappeared entirely, never to return. This time, it was not a neurosis which I had in place of them, nor was it a new life and a neurosis, but just the new life without any neurosis, the new life in place of neurosis and neuralgia.

It could be said that my compulsive researches and quest for knowledge were symptomatic of some restless drive, some potentially morbid compulsion. The answer is, of course, that so long as they were not frustrated, so long as I could pursue these interests freely, without interference from environment or from intrapsychic conflict such as worry or anxiety, while this movement, however compulsive, could continue, I was well. In the same way, we might say that so long as a man or any animal is allowed to move and behave according to his impulses, we do not say he is morbid because he has these impulses; we might even suggest he were morbid if he had not, but certainly, if an animal such as a dog wants to run about and research round the lamp posts and elsewhere, we may say that he is well, although he is engaging himself in these activities. He might not be well if the activities were stopped and he were not allowed to use his inherited skeletal muscles. His health would deteriorate unless he could be perpetually repeating the inherited instinct drives and compulsions acquired, developed and passed on by his ancestors. These are represented in him both physically (e.g. in his possession of the same skeletal muscles as his ancestors) and psychologically.

It is part of the nature of life to have such things, just as it was part of the nature of my life, no doubt fundamentally inherited, to have the compulsions which I had and which, in some form and degree, are common to all living things.

Now I was using them and thereby keeping my mental tensions, both in their intellectual and emotional forms, within normal and healthy limits. I have no doubt this is the basis not only of happiness, but of health and of life itself. This is true whether it be a fetish we are following or any other emotional pattern or compulsion. Indeed, it is doubtful whether life, the behaviour of life, consists of much else except the utilisation of realities around us as toys with which to play out afresh the old games, the games or reactions of our ancestors and of our infancy, in these seemingly new forms. We can see it in insects, birds and fishes, and with psychoanalytical help we can see it in ourselves, in our activities and emotions and in our very habits of thought and belief. We do not choose, that is an illusion, albeit one that is very dear to us; we are driven by the past, ancestral and infantile, driven and lived by the life forces and patterns which gave rise to us, which formed us as we are and which continue to express themselves through us and to make us lend ourselves unwittingly to their expression.

CHAPTER XVIII

HAPPINESS AND RELAXATION

IT is a curious reflection that when the subject matter is 'happiness', we have nothing to write about. 'They lived happily ever after' is the end of every story—or fairy tale(!)—never the beginning. It is the equivalent of the Buddhists' 'Nirvana' (Nothingness), which may sound to us more depressing than exhilarating. My patient who says that when everything is calm and quiet he 'feels like death', feels that, if no one else will do so, *he* has to 'start something up'—an argument, or anything, 'to get a bit of life into things'. Incidentally he is the patient I previously mentioned whose home environment in his childhood was a continuous row between each member of the household, mother and father, brothers and sisters. He feels lost unless there is a hullabaloo going on. If nobody else will start it, he must. The process, or the initial movement, is commonly unconscious.

We may reflect that if a play were put upon the stage that excluded all such elements, if it depicted shall we say just Darby and Joan sitting peacefully and happily each side of the fireplace, it would not be long before the audience yawned and walked out of the theatre! Does this mean that, like this patient, we all have within us reactive patterns of some age-old battle or struggle for existence, and that we demand that these reactive patterns shall be perenially stimulated, to keep our life-processes moving? If so, what is this quietude or rest or happiness which we are alleged to be seeking?

My answer is that what we are seeking is a freedom from environmental frustrations, so that we can indulge ourselves in our particular individual battle-patterns, and in our projection of them on to an acquiescent environment; or, better, an environment which will respond to and accept the roles which our unconscious drama would fain thrust upon it. This is the process, the only process, whereby we can get relief from our internal tensions, the tensions provoked by the struggle for existence, the battle of the ages, which has gone on inside us and received some characteristic individual pattern during our babyhood, infancy and growth. When we speak of relaxation or of happiness, we are speaking of a situation or environment which will permit us 'to be ourselves', which will not interfere with our re-living our individual battle-pattern in phantasy or in fact. That is what we mean by relaxation as a prerequisite for health and happiness.

Relaxation is essential, not only at the analytical session, but in general for any healthy intra-psychic movement or adjustment to take place. Probably we have enough conflicts and disturbances going on within us in the deeper and unconscious levels, remnants of our past, particularly of our infancy, to be able to do very much with present-day realities other than to play out these conflicts, to live them out again, in the environment of these realities, using the realities as 'props' for our necessary psychodrama. Of course, we do not know that we are doing this. We think erroneously that we are reacting appropriately to the realities around us at the time; but *analysis shows that what we are doing is compulsively repeating the emotional patterns of our past, dating right back to infancy and earlier, and merely manipulating the things and persons around us in order to facilitate our acting out of the tensions belonging to these unconscious repressed patterns and complexes of ours.*

If the environment, if realities about us do not permit us to do these things, then they are, as it were, frustrating us, beating us up, interfering with our health-giving 'game'. It is then that reality, now an uncongenial, impossible environment, seems to be making us ill. It is making us ill, not necessarily by any activity on its part, but merely by its being a barrier or frustration to our need to play out our compulsions and tensions, our necessity to use it as a prop in our tension-relieving psychodrama. If the environment is not interfering, indeed if there is no appreciable environment present (if one could imagine such a thing), there is at least nothing to impede us; we go on working out the tensions of our emotional patterns in dreams and phantasies, conscious and unconscious. We may protest a little that we have no props, no reality, to assist us in dramatising our nature, in expressing and relieving the tension of the complexes that lie within us, like a child may protest at having no toys with which to play his games.

I have inadvertently expressed in a few careless paragraphs

the profoundest and most far-reaching discovery of clinical analysis, expecting the reader to swallow it whole, presenting him with scarcely a sample of the evidence upon which this statement is founded. I imagine this has happened simply because it is my professional experience every day and all day with all patients. Relaxing and doing free association of thought, this experience consists essentially in hearing people repeating the emotional experiences, the drama, of their infancy and early childhood again and again, *clad in the clothing of their present-day circumstances*, the old story edited anew, or retold with up-to-date people and things in the role of those who once comprised their early environment—like Shakespeare played in modern dress and in modern life.

The emotional reaction patterns set up or reinforced in a living creature during the earliest and most impressionable and malleable weeks, months and years of its life after birth (as well as before it) should, in the light of clinical experience, to my mind, be looked upon as an 'acquired instinct'. Of course, I know that the expression is a contradiction in terms, a flagrant contradiction, but in the same way as I would define an instinct as 'a phylogenetically acquired reflex' so have I equal justification for regarding these reaction patterns acquired by very early emotional experiences, and so irradicable throughout the individual's life, as tantamount to 'acquired instincts'. Their nature, and their mode of creation and development, are identical. This theory is, to my mind, in itself a justification for the writing of this book. In spite of modern biological theory and its concentration on ancillary mechanisms (orthodox theory has been consistently wrong in the pre-Darwinian Past), *my clinical analytical experience* proves to me that the essential process in evolution, and in life and survival, is *adaptation*, and, eventually, transmissible adaptation (e.g. instincts) neo-Lamarckianwise.

Thus, reflexes, conditioned reflexes, instincts, and emotional reactive patterns, inherited and acquired, are all different stages of natural nervous reaction to stimuli, environmental and endogenous. They are only special instances of the general reaction of living matter to forces which impinge upon it, from without and from within, and are of the very nature and essence of living matter and of the life-process which enables it to continue to live;

in short, adaptation. The only differences between them are differences of the stage of evolution or development at which the particular form of reaction was acquired. The earliest 'reflexes' were probably as early as unicellular life, and certainly as early as the first nervous tissue or even the neuromuscular bands of paramecium. Instincts are a later and more elaborate combination of established reflexes and acquired reactive patterns. Later combinations of this sort are the precursors of *later* instincts, actually in the making, and often too young to be as yet transmissible to offspring, but nevertheless precursors of a potential phylogenetic modification, being formed in just the same way as inherited reflexes and instincts were originally formed. This is a sample of the essential dynamics of the living process, adaptation and evolution.

These patterns, these reactive emotional patterns, inherited or acquired, undoubtedly tend to order and direct our lives from their inception to our demise. We cling to the precious illusion of free will, but the truth, revealed by science, is that *we are lived by these life-forces* in accordance with their reactive nature, inherited and acquired. In ordinary life, we project our unconscious emotional patterns, positive and negative, upon others, and they project their emotional patterns, positive and negative, upon us. The only essential difference between this state of emotional personal relationship and that prevailing in the analytical situation is that in the former, the family and social situation, nobody has any insight, very often one has not any insight oneself, into the source and mechanism of what is going on. On the other hand, in the analytical situation the minds of analyst and, through him, of patient are concentrated upon insight, and it is only through insight that anything other than havoc will result. If one were a god or even a son of god (i.e. completely cured oneself) these extra-analytical relationships would be all right, a triumph of psychology for all to see. Unfortunately one is not a god, nor even a son of god, and therefore outside the consulting room, off duty, one is only too apt to regress, at least temporarily, to the usual, primitive emotional levels without insight and not without the familiar diastrous results that spell havoc and are the basis of the drama, the comedy and the tragedy, of human life, familially, socially, nationally and internationally.

In the analytical session, through relaxation and free association of thought, one is naturally giving expression to all these intra-psychic matters in a verbal form, one is speaking them all aloud, writing the script, as it were, of one's psychodrama while the analyst listens. Maybe from a gratification point of view, this is the next best thing to acting it out in the real world. From the point of view of insight and conscious appreciation of what we are doing, it is, of course, infinitely better than acting it out in the real world. Everybody is engaged all the time in acting it out in the real world, and probably by that very fact, he or she is avoiding insight instead of getting it; but, provided one can continue to act it out successfully, one maintains an optimum or tolerable level of tension, homeostasis, or relaxation within oneself, and that is what we call mental and emotional health—however disastrous it may be to our personal relationships, in the family, in society, in the community and in the world.

L'ENVOI.

Now the time at Polzeath has come to an end. I have tried to follow the principle that I insist upon in my patients under analysis, namely, that they should relax and give the habit of editing their thoughts and words a holiday. I have noticed that they become interesting immediately they cease to edit. If I have bored you, it is because I have failed to be quite natural. That would not be surprising in view of the life-long training we all received. It is a pity because nature is the ultimate criterion of the true and the good.

I have found it very pleasant to talk out my thoughts in this large and lovely meadow, sloping down to the cliff overlooking the bay. This four or five hours dictating to my long-suffering secretary, every morning between breakfast and lunch, for three weeks, has resulted in so many hundreds of thousands of words that it is obvious that the resulting manuscript will have to be cut down to less than half its length. Now the time has come to an end, and I am looking forward to returning to my patients with anticipation and interest. What am I doing, or rather what is being done to me? I am doing, or being driven to do, what I have always done,

what has always been done to me; I am being diverted by a spontaneous, *compulsive*, interest from the practical and the 'relevant'
order of things to absorption in what may be called my 'addiction'!
Perhaps it is not so irrelevant. It is the very essence of all that
has happened to me. I will give you a typical little anecdote to
illustrate what I mean.

Only a few weeks ago at the Psychiatric Hospital where I work,
it was seven o'clock and time that I left to go home. At home
there awaited me a long-suffering wife . . . and on this occasion,
of all things, a dinner party! I knew it. Therefore, when the
last patient proved to be a newcomer, I swore a bit inwardly, felt
some resistance to listening to his problem, to becoming absorbed
in it and having to solve it. In my experience, nervous disorders
commonly prove to be a person's whole-life problem, and it is
impossible to do justice to such a protracted subject if one is in
a hurry. I was silently wondering how I could deal with the
impossible situation.

In the meantime, the patient had plunged into a recital of his
symptoms. The more he talked, the more complicated and intriguing became the problem of his illness. It was not long before there
appeared to be nothing in the universe except this man, his fears
and his hopes, and his potentially solvable problem. Listening,
as his nature and character increasingly revealed themselves, I
found myself becoming as usual fascinated at the unsuspected
relevance of his personality as a factor in the production of his
illness. An intriguing problem always at the back of one's mind
is how one is going to deal with characterological obstacles to
improvement. It was early in the interview that I glanced at the
clock. When I next looked at it, another half-hour had passed.
Dinner parties! I had quite forgotten that there were such things—
and this in the presence of what might be regarded as a typical,
mediocre and commonplace type of case!

Therefore I say, these case digressions on the very last pages
of this book about my life are, in fact, not digressions at all. They
serve to illustrate the answers to the main problems with which the
book is concerned. The first is why my life became what it has
become, and the second why my philosophy, why all philosophy,
leaves The Riddle unsolved. As regards the first, I would possibly
be of even inferior value in my particular branch of the profession

were it not for this 'unpractical' (?) addiction that posseses me and compels. I would add that the same curiosity-ridden 'addiction' which compels me to try to unravel a person's psychopathology, to trace the causes from the clues, also prompts me, with only less compulsive force, to try to unravel the causes both of social behaviour and of cosmic behaviour. It is inadequately described by the alleged attribute of 'having an enquiring mind'. It is something more compulsive than that. Perhaps I shall have to call it an 'addiction'.

I am reminded of an unusual patient, a hair fetishist. He presented himself for treatment because he was a man with the ideal of being a perfect husband to his wife and a perfect father to his children. But ideals or no ideals, it made very little difference. He had only to see a woman with a particular type of coiffure and he was in the throes of a struggle which sometimes led to his being compelled to follow her for hours, suffering agonies of conflict on account of his duty to get home at the expected time, and yet feeling powerless to resist what was, at instinct level, a stronger compulsion than those of home, family and civilisation. In so far as this man was inhibited or frustrated from following this perversion, to that degree did he suffer from an acute Anxiety State with all its intolerable symptoms, including tremor, palpitation and giddiness, and even gastric pain. The compulsion or addiction absorbed the energy that otherwise went into anxiety. One has to study such cases closely to appreciate the power of the force involved. It is the compulsion of life itself.

I am more fortunate in the *form* of my particular addiction; but let us put all emphasis on the word 'fortunate'. Should we take credit or discredit for being born a spider, a rabbit, or a particular type of human being? Admittedly our fate may be decided by our 'fortune'. When one studies the family history or the chronological 'family tree' of some unfortunate neurotic sufferer, psychopath, epileptic or criminal, one sees the black-marked eccentric and mentally-ill personalities that have added up Mendelian-wise into our particular black sheep.

As regards my second problem, these cases, and some others which I could mention, help to indicate to the unbiased analyst that 'revelations', like those contained in this book, whether they come from the divesting of clothes, material or mental, or from the deepest analysis that can be achieved, are not necessarily a complete or a sufficient answer.

What is, what would be or could be a sufficient answer? I think we will come nearest to a complete answer when we can precisely correlate psychological changes with chemico-physical processes. Even Freud said somewhere that psychological problems must eventually become physiological problems. Alexander, the Chicago analyst, has underlined it. Thus we will get an intellectually 'satisfactory' answer (and perhaps satisfaction is by its very nature a matter of degree) only when we know the very chemistry of thought. We do not seem to be very near it at present.

If my carefree book has intrigued and interested you, perhaps we should both be satisfied—at least to some degree! I have tried to be natural and genuine. Anyhow that is all I can do, maybe it is all anybody can do, and all he can claim to do if he is honest.

GLOSSARY

Aetiology. The science of causation.

Affect. The energy of an emotion. See *Displacement.*

Analysand. One who is being treated by analysis.

Anamnesis. Detailed history from the earliest memory.

Clinical. Originally of or pertaining to the sick-bed and hence to do with observation of the actual patient, as distinct from theoretical constructions.

Complex. A group of affectively charged ideas which, through conflict, have become repressed into the unconscious.

Component Instinct. See *Libidinal Organisation.*

Conflict. 'War' between opposing elements in the mind.

Cyclothymia. A condition characterised by recurring phases of elation and depression, its extreme form being manic-depressive psychosis.

Death Instinct. A deeply rooted instinctual impulse that tends to take the organism back as far as possible to its original inorganic state. It is supposed to be closely associated with destructive, aggressive and repetitive tendencies in the psyche, and to contrast with the 'life' or libidinal instinct.

Defence Resistance. All contrivances, conscious and unconscious, employed by a person to avoid insight into his motivations, and specifically by an analysand to retard the progress of his analysis.

Dementia Praecox. See *Schizophrenia.*

Detumescence. A term much used by Havelock Ellis to denote orgasm or subsidence of sexual tumidity. See *Tumescence.*

Displacement. The transfer of an affect from the idea to which it was originally attached to an associated idea. It is one of the most important unconscious mechanisms in the production of phobias and other symptoms.

Ego. That part of the id which has become modified by the impingement of external stimuli in such a way that it has become adapted to reality, reality testing and activity, and is credited with consciousness. In contradistinction to the id, it tends to organisation into a united whole.

Erotic. Sexual.

Erotogenic Zones. Sensitive areas of the body stimulation of which gives rise to erotic feelings. These areas are often where mucous membranes join skin at the bodily orifices.

Euphoria. A sense of well-being, usually morbid or abnormal.

Extravert. One who turns his interests outward and experiences his emotional life in relation to the stimuli of the external world.

Fetish. Anything which is attractive on account of its association, usually through unconscious elements, with erotic pleasure.

Fixation. Arrest of a portion of the libidinal stream at an immature stage of development, either with reference to its erotogenic zone or with reference to its object attachment or both. The level of a fixation determines the type of any psychosis or psychoneurosis which later may occur, and the nature of its object attachment may determine its presenting form.

Frigidity. Absence of normal sexual desire and response, especially in women.

Frustration. The action of frustrating, or an obstacle or force which stands in the way of gratification or of the aim of an instinct.

Genital Organisation. The mature stage of libidinal development. In infancy it gives rise to the Oedipus complex and in later life to psychosexual union. And see *Libidinal Organisation.*

Heterosexuality. Love for or erotic interest in a person of the opposite sex, *i.e.* normal psychosexual development.

Homosexuality. Sexual desire for a member of the same sex.

Hypochondria or Hypochondriasis. A condition or morbid anxiety about the health, in which various healthy organs are believed to be diseased.

Hysteria. A psychoneurotic disorder resulting from a conflict between the libido, including non-genital organisation thereof, and the ego or super-ego, in which the libidinal drives are repressed and thus excluded from direct or conscious expression, and in which the unconscious repressed material later, through displacement and conversion, finds an outlet by an indirect somatic pathway and thus produces symptoms. Freud described two principal varieties: (1) anxiety hysteria, in which the predominating symptom is anxiety but distinguishable from anxiety neurosis in that the aetiological factors are psychological (such as infantile sexual traumata) rather than physical (e.g. disturbances in the current sex life); and (2) conversion hysteria, in which the principal symptoms are physical (hysterical pains, visceral disturbances, paralyses, etc.).

Id. The concept of an undifferentiated primitive mind containing only innate urges, instincts, desires and wishes without consciousness or any appreciation of reality, and apparently dominated by the pleasure-pain principle. Unlike the ego it is not organised or integrated, so that contrary and incompatible urges can exist side by side in it without necessarily entering into conflict with each other.

Imago. The fantastic image formed in infancy from an erroneous conception of a loved or hated person.

Impotence. Psychosexual impotence: inability on the part of the male to perform the normal heterosexual act. (Minor degrees of impotence are commonly unrecognised).

Infantile Amnesia. The memory blank which obscures the adult's recollection of periods of his infancy.

Inhibition. Restraint of an impulse by an opposing intra-psychic force. A frustration from within the psyche.

Instincts. Innate patterns of discharge of tension.

Introjection. A process of 'assimilation' of an object (e.g. a person) and of feelings associated to it or him, whereas 'projection' is a process of dissimilation.

Introversion. The reversal of the libidinal stream from outward-seeking to inward-absorption, with consequent withdrawal of interest from the external world to the internal world of self. When extreme in degree it is one of the characteristics of schizophrenia, melancholia, hypo-chondriasis, etc.

Libidinal Organisation. The emotional pattern or system of sequences assumed by the libido. The libido passes through many stages in the course of development. From oral to genital the component instincts all have their own organisation or pattern, but full maturity is reached only at the genital level of libidinal organisation with its whole-object (persons as such) relationship.

Libido. The energy of the sexual instinct and of its psychosexual component instincts. It is subject to many vicissitudes. For example, it can become aim-inhibited (*i.e.* orgasm-inhibited) and undergo unlimited displacement, even on to the person's own ego (narcissism, self-love), asexual objects and abstract ideas.

Manic. Pertaining to mania, or the exalted phase of manic-depressive psychosis.

Manic-Depressive Psychosis. A well-defined psychosis of the affective group characterised by (1) elation with over-activity, or (2) depression with psychomotor retardation, or (3) mixed forms. It usually remits, though chronic states can supervene, and it is not so prone to lead to dementia as are other psychoses.

Masochism. Erotic pleasure in being victimised or hurt (cf. *Sadism*).

Neurosis. A functional nervous disorder. By some writers used to designate any psychogenic illness.

Obsessional Neurosis. A psychoneurosis characterised by the presence of obsessions which dominate the thought processes and behaviour of the patient. Compulsion neurosis.

Oedipus Complex. According to Freud the most important complex belonging to the period of infantile amnesia. It coincides with the arrival of genital organisation of the libido. At this stage of development (about three years of age) infantile phantasy possesses the parent of the opposite sex after the same pattern as the phantasy of the suckling infant possesses the mother's nipple or breast. But one of the difficulties of this latter complex is that it is accompanied by the phantasy of liquidating all opposition which eventually takes the form of the rival parent of the same sex. Fear, guilt and renunciation supervene. There appears to be evidence of this surprising structure of the primitive mind not only in the unconscious of every adult, but also in anthropological and social patterns of behaviour.

Ontogenesis. Development of the individual.

Oral Erotism. Erotic excitation from stimulation of the mouth or lips, the primary source of erotic feelings in babyhood and continuing in variable degree throughout life in spite of the acquisition of genital maturity with which it becomes associated, as evidenced by the phenomena of kissing and various habits and perversions.

Orgasm. The point at which erotic excitement reaches its acme and becomes involuntary. On the latter account it is disordered or suppressed by most persons in proportion to their prevailing anxiety and ill-health.

Orgastic Potency. The degree of capacity to achieve 'perfect' orgasm, that is to say an orgasm which will result in complete reduction of sexual tension and at the same time satisfy the whole psyche, i.e. without residual disturbance or conflict.

Paranoia. A psychosis characterised by systematised delusions commonly of persecution, love or hate. Freud considers that it has its source in repressed (unconscious) homosexual desires.

Parent Surrogate. A substitute for the parent, often not recognised as such.

Part-objects. Anatomical parts of a person which may be objects of intense love or hate without reference to the person as a whole. For instance, the baby loves the breast or nipple (a part-object) without necessarily his mother as a 'whole-object'. The persistence of this tendency into adult life is a measure of various libidinal fixations. Cf. *Fetish.*

Perversion. Any sexual act the object or mechanism of which is both biologically unsound and socially disapproved. Perversions are usually the manifestation of a psychosexual component instinct in substitution for mature genital sexuality. Their development is encouraged by frustration of the latter.

Phobia. Morbid or unjustifiable fear, e.g. of some harmless object, activity or situation. It is unconsciously associated with some repressed and feared instinct desire.

Phylogenesis. Biogenic development or evolution, e.g. of race or species. (Cf. *Ontogenesis*: the development of the individual).

Pre-genital Sexuality. The infantile organisation of the sexual pattern in which the component instincts and the pre-genital erotogenic zones, such as oral, anal, urethral and phallic, are absorbing the greater part of the libido.

Projection. The attributing to persons or things outside oneself of mental processes, affects, etc., that originated within one's own mind (and have been repressed), with relief of tension; common in varying degrees to all minds, with consequent impairment of their reality appreciation. It is very characteristic of paranoia and of the finding of scapegoats. (Cf. *Introjection.*)

Psyche. Mind.

Psychiatry. That branch of medical science which deals with mental diseases and disorders.

Psychoanalysis. (1) A technical method introduced by Freud of bringing unconscious conflicts, complexes, etc., into consciousness by the process of free association of thought, dream analysis and interpretation of the transference situation. (2) The body of knowledge so obtained, including its theoretical interpretation.

Psychogenic. Originating in the mind.

Psychoneurosis. Psychogenic illness (i.e. without organic cause) characterised by derangement of the normal ways of gratification of the libido due to unconscious conflict, and, while leaving the ego or reason relatively unimpaired (cf. *Psychosis*), giving rise to a variety of symptoms and pathological states which are amenable to psychotherapy.

Psychosis. Insanity. Mental illness which includes the ego or reason and therefore the person's relationship to reality. (Cf. *Psychoneurosis*).

Psychotic. Mad. (Adjective of psychosis).

Psychotherapy. The treatment of psychoneurotic, characterological and psychotic disorders by psychological methods, usually one of the forms of mind analysis, or by explanation, persuasion, re-education, relaxation, suggestion, hypnosis, vegetotherapy (Reich) or by occupational therapy.

Rationalisation. The attributing of reasons for judgments, ideas or actions which are otherwise (usually emotionally) determined.

Reaction Formation. A character trait, or its development, unconsciously designed to hold in check, conceal or contradict a tendency of an opposite kind. Thus obsessional cleanliness would be a reaction formation against repressed dirtying tendencies. Disgust, shame and morality are other reaction formations.

Reactive pattern. A form of reaction based on instinct, but acquired by the individual at an early stage of his development and tending to be repeated (like instincts) throughout his life.

Regression. The reversal of the normal direction of the libidinal stream so that early infantile stages of its development (fixation points) are reactivated.

Repression. The rejection from consciousness, by an unconscious mechanism, of mental material, concepts and affects, which are unwelcome. Analysis has shown that this material remains active, and dynamic in the unconscious, that the expenditure of repressing energy continues and that the repressed commonly re-emerges in altered forms such as symptoms.

Sadism. The achievement of erotic pleasure by victimising the sexual object, commonly by inflicting helplessness or pain upon him or her. (Cf. *Masochism*).

Schizophrenia. Split mind. A psychosis, usually in early life, characterised by repressed affect, introversion, withdrawal of interest, and progressive dementia in the absence of remissions.

Screen Memories. Memories which by carrying the affects of some earlier experience serve to relieve to some extent the tension of that experience and thereby to cover, or inhibit, its emergence into consciousness.

Sublimation. The process of deflecting libido from sexual aims to interests of a non-sexual and socially approved nature.

Superego. That part of the mental apparatus developed in early life by the mechanism of repressing frustrated impulses, such as aggression, and projecting them on the frustrators (e.g. parents) and subsequently introjecting them. Its function is largely to oppose the id, often unreasonably, and even to criticise and punish the ego if it tends to accept id demands. It is a sort of primitive unconscious conscience, formed largely from parent-imagos.

Syndrome. A group of symptoms or signs which are found together and appear to form a clinical entity, but which, in the absence of the discovery of a common underlying cause, cannot be held to constitute a disease entity.

Transference. A displacement of any affect from one person to another. Specifically during analysis the affects originally felt during infancy for the parents become unconsciously displaced on to the person of the analyst so that the analysand feels towards him unjustifiable love and hate and has no insight into the phenomenon and its irrelevance.

Transference Resistance. The resistance which an analysand exhibits to the normal analytical process of transferring his infant-parent affects on to the image of his analyst. At the same time it should be borne in mind that the phenomenon of transference is itself a resistance to the memories of the childhood emotions which were originally experienced during the Oedipus situation.

Trigeminal Neuralgia. Tic douloureux. Neuralgia (pain) in one or more of the three branches of the trigeminal or fifth cranial nerve. The sensory branches of this nerve supply the skin over the forehead and front of the scalp, around the eye, the cheek, the upper and lower jaws, the teeth, tongue and the interior of the mouth and throat. The pain can be incredibly severe, sometimes causing a spasm of muscles in the affected region. It is usually psychoneurotic in origin.

Tumescence. A swelling-up. Specifically the turgidity produced in the sexual organs during the pre-orgasm stage of sexual excitement.

Unconscious. A region of the psyche which contains mental proccesses and constellations which are ordinarily inaccessible to consciousness, commonly owing to the process of repression. The technique of mind analysis is especially designed to bring this unconscious material into consciousness by overcoming the resistances and repressing forces. It is from the unconscious conflicts or complexes and their opposing forces or reaction formations that all symptoms emanate.

Whole-objects. The person as a whole, in contradistinction to exclusive interest in some anatomical part. (Cf. *Part-objects*).

For Product Safety Concerns and Information please contact our EU
representative GPSR@taylorandfrancis.com
Taylor & Francis Verlag GmbH, Kaufingerstraße 24, 80331 München, Germany